"*When All Becomes New* is a rare and soul of a man tasked with 'cavorting b a neonatologist. Each beautifully draw nating collection explores the gut-wren........ gate of emotions Dr. Rattray must grapple with during even the most routine NICU moments. Full of empathy and honesty, this book is ultimately a spiritual journey punctuated with anguish, deep human connection, joy, perspective, and ultimately, reconciliation. It is a story that will surely cast hope and heal hearts."

—CARRIE FIRESTONE
Author of *The Unlikelies*

"This book is pure treasure. It is rare to get a realistic glimpse into the world of medicine. Dr. Rattray has been able to not only provide that glimpse, but also to combine it with the thoughts and emotions that all of us called to practice medicine experience. His humble, picturesque prose will take you deep into the heart and soul of the art of medicine. From the heartwarming success stories to the devastating loss of a life not yet begun, it will be impossible to read without the stirring of deep emotions. This book should be required reading for anyone considering a career in medicine. Fantastic!"

—MICHAEL R. CANADY
Chief Executive Officer, Holzer Health System, Gallipolis, Ohio

"The stories of the families in the NICU are masterfully interwoven with Dr. Rattray's reflections on the journey of his own young family. Written with heart and raw honesty, this book bridges the invisible barrier between physician and patient. I highly recommend this book, although I caution that it is almost impossible to put down once you start."

—ALANA LEDFORD
Communications Professor

"Have you ever wondered about what goes on in a NICU? Wonder no more, as Ben Rattray has written a must-read of vivid, true stories about what happens inside the doors of a world that many will never enter."

—CHRIS ROWE
Neonatal Nurse Practitioner

"*When All Becomes New* is a beautiful unification of perspective—the untouchable medical profession with the realness of actuality. Dr. Rattray allows us the unique gift of peeking inside the world of a physician, in the often-hidden specialty of neonatal medicine. His stories highlight his evolution from young courage to a foundation of steadfast faith that is tangible within the pages. The stories are raw, some even unimaginable, yet throughout the beauty of their realness there is an intertwining of Dr. Rattray's fundamental framework, his deepest calling—that of grace that can only be attributed to his love for the Lord."

—KATIE KRIST
Neonatal Nurse Practitioner

"*When All Becomes New* captures the compassion and love Dr. Rattray shares with his newborn patients and their parents, inviting the reader into a place of gentleness and wonder. Before reading this book, I knew little of neonatology; afterwards I had a far deeper appreciation for the nuances of this area of medicine. Dr. Rattray humanizes his discipline, inviting the reader into the exhilaration and joy of new life taking hold or the tragedy of it being extinguished before it's even begun. He captures the fragility of premature infants tenuously balancing between life and death. Seemingly simple things in adults, like placing intravenous lines or breathing tubes, become harrowing life-and-death challenges in a tiny baby. He honors and remembers his losses yet delights in meeting his young patients who have gone on to grow into healthy and happy children. Dr. Rattray interweaves vignettes from his own life—his marriage, his training, his faith, his own children—with tender, captivating, compelling stories from his days and nights as guardian of the NICU."

—JOSEPH STERN
Author of *Grief Connects Us: A Neurosurgeon's Lessons on Love, Loss, and Compassion*

"When you flip to the prologue of a book and read, "The baby's heart rate suddenly disappears from the monitor . . . ," you absolutely must, no matter how tired you are, keep reading, mustn't you? *When All Becomes New* offers readers a glimpse behind the curtain of the NICU. But this is not just a rehash of something you might have watched during the heyday of must-see TV. Rattray invites us into the private thoughts and life of a neonatal physician, a life where he struggles to preserve the 'humanity in medicine drowned under the weight of fatigue, stress, and a crushing workload'—and, in doing so, he has given us a book that, in some ways, we wish had never been written, while also being moved by its empathy and compassion."

—**TERRY L. KENNEDY**
Editor, *The Greensboro Review*

"*When All Becomes New* is a poignant, heart-wrenching, and heart-warming intersection of Dr. Rattray's chosen path in pediatric neonatology and life beyond profession as a father, husband, and son. His prose will capture you just as swiftly as the tales from life tending to the littlest inhabitants of the pediatric neonatology unit. Each one of them touches his heart and will touch yours as well. Each story illuminates the soulful battle Dr. Rattray faces daily as he deftly weaves the calling of a life in medicine with his own spiritual journey. This story will leave you humbled, awed, healed, and inspired."

—**JADE MCCARTHY**
TV personality, writer, speaker

"*When All Becomes New* offers a wonderfully riveting behind-the-scenes look at life in the NICU, told through dozens of stories from throughout Dr. Rattray's career.
Not only does Dr. Rattray provide gripping play-by-play accounts of what transpires, but he also offers candid perspectives on the mental, physical, and emotional implications of these cases on medical-care professionals, patients, and families. Through stories of incredible successes and tragic outcomes, Dr. Rattray unabashedly explores the roles of training, intuition, randomness, and faith on life and death, and shares personal perspectives on the meanings behind it all."

—**AYDIN KADASTER**
Managing Director, Revyrie, and Founder, Kadaster Ventures

When All Becomes New

When All Becomes New

A Doctor's Stories of Life, Love, and Loss

Benjamin Rattray

RESOURCE *Publications* · Eugene, Oregon

WHEN ALL BECOMES NEW
A Doctor's Stories of Life, Love, and Loss

Resource Publications
An Imprint of Wipf and Stock Publishers
199 W. 8th Ave., Suite 3
Eugene, OR 97401

www.wipfandstock.com

PAPERBACK ISBN: 978-1-6667-0490-7
HARDCOVER ISBN: 978-1-6667-0491-4
EBOOK ISBN: 978-1-6667-0492-1

08/12/21

for
Danielle
and for Owen, Hannah, and Avery

. . . 'Behold, the dwelling of God is with men. He will dwell with them, and they shall be his people, and God himself will be with them; **4**he will wipe away every tear from their eyes, and death shall be no more, neither shall there be mourning nor crying nor pain any more, for the former things have passed away.'

5And he who sat upon the throne said, 'Behold, I make all things new.'

REVELATION 21:3–5 (RSV)

Contents

Acknowledgements

This book is twenty years in the making, from the time a college friend handed me her father's book of patient stories until now. I am deeply grateful to all those who have shaped this journey.

To my parents, Maggie and Stuart, for pouring into me and modeling compassion, thoughtfulness and how to love others. To my sister Alana for your enthusiastic pride in your big brother despite how I shoved you in that hole and super-glued things to your desk. To Mike and Jeanette Kyser, who have never fit the definition of in-laws and who, like your daughter, have always believed in me. To my daughters, Hannah and Avery, and my son Owen, for enduring dinner conversations about Tim O'Brien and polysyndeton and for always being my biggest fans. You are my world. To my wife, Danielle, for your steadfast confidence, your beauty of character, and your love.

To all those who taught and mentored me—you not only introduced me to medical literature, you invested heavily in me over those formative years of college, medical school, and training. I will forever be grateful to Dr. Ronald Goldberg, my fellowship program director, who mentored and guided me throughout my training. Your support meant the world to me and yes, Danielle is feeding me enough. I am indebted to all those at Duke University Medical Center who taught me invaluable lessons—you know who you are, so thank you.

To my neonatology colleagues, nurse practitioners, nurses, and caregivers whom I am fortunate enough to work alongside every day—you are a bedrock for the babies and their families. You have lived through many of these stories and they are your own as well.

Acknowledgements

To those who helped these stories become a book—Maureen Tobin, you pushed me to go deeper and find the true story; your guidance is woven into these chapters. Thank you, Irene Connelly, for your sharp editorial eye and insights. To Terry Kennedy who agreed to a cup of coffee and ended up helping me launch a hospital writing program. Thank you, Cynthia Nearman, Emilia Philips, Mike Gaspeny, and Jessie Van Rheenen, for lending your MFA teaching skills and wisdom. And to my colleagues in the provider writing group who helped me work through many thoughts and ideas. To Carrie Firestone, you were the first author to read a chapter and offer your generous encouragement and advice. To the early readers, Chris Rowe, Alana Ledford, and Katie Krist, thank you for spending time with those early drafts. To Victoria Pryor, for your unswerving belief in this book. To Tim Blocker, for showing me a new way of seeing things. To everyone at Wipf and Stock for putting these black lines on the page.

I am deeply grateful to my patients and to the families who allow me into their lives during their most intense times of joy and suffering.

Note

These pages contain an anthology of true stories. I have changed identifying information to protect patient confidentiality, except in a few instances when the family gave permission to use their names. The details are as true as I can remember based on my observations and interactions except for intentional changes in immaterial details to preserve privacy. Any error in the telling is mine.

Prologue

T he baby's heart rate suddenly disappears from the monitor and when I listen, there is nothing.

I stand over baby Olivia in Room 5 at the bed closest to the window. Her skin is ashen, cool, and rubbery like dough, her face expressionless and peaceful. All I can think about is taking the elevator to her mother's room and telling the parents that their baby is dead.

"Laurie, can you start compressions? Can someone get epi?" I call out.

"She's about fourteen hundred grams so let's give her point four milliliters of epi. Is someone charting this?"

I push the drops of epinephrine into the IV while the nurse counts out the compressions, squeezing her thumbs into the baby's pliant sternum. Three minutes later I give another dose of epinephrine and when I listen, there is a faint thrumming. She is alive.

On the X-ray, the left side of her chest is black where the lung has collapsed and her heart is shoved to the right from the pleural air. An emergency chest tube: swabs of muddy betadine, the sickening lurch as the curved forceps pop through the lung pleura, and the satisfying hiss of air released. The oxygen saturation monitor starts picking up and she shifts under the drape. I watch the intermittent misting of the chest tube; the blue water of the canister bubbles and her saturations climb steadily. Relief rises in my chest and I take a deep breath. I look over at her nurse, Laurie, and she smiles under her mask, her eyes creased at the corners.

That evening I pull into the garage and as I open the mudroom door, my daughters run up to me, bouncing up and down. "Daddy, you're home!"

I drop my worn leather bag between a pair of pink cowgirl boots and a purple backpack, bending down to hug my girls.

"Hey babe," my wife calls out from the kitchen. She is juggling cooking and helping our daughters with homework. The countertop is covered with dishes, school papers, crayons, and hundreds of little pieces of cut-up paper.

I kiss her hello, thinking of how lovely she looks, and head upstairs to wash my face and change. With the hot water running I splash my face, rub soap into my stinging eyes, and imagine myself washing away the day. I am home and I resume my role as a father and husband. Twelve miles south, within the walls of the hospital, everything will continue as it always does, twenty-four hours a day, seven days a week.

"Honey, dinner's ready," my wife calls up the stairs.

At the table Avery, my youngest daughter, offers thanks for the day's blessings.

"Dad, how was your day?" my son Owen asks.

"Did you send any babies home?" my daughter Hannah asks before I can answer.

Out the window the evening sun hits the tops of the pines and the trees sway slowly into each other; the grass is a patchwork of shadow and light and my eye catches the area by the crepe myrtle where the grass is thin and sparse.

"It was okay," I say, giving my wife a look that tells a different story. "One of the babies got a little sick but I think she'll be fine. We did have two babies go home, though."

Avery squeals and claps her hands, sending Parmesan cheese crumbs flying.

"I love it when babies go home," she says.

"I do too, sweetie," I reply.

So many years have passed since I first entered the neonatal intensive care unit. But even now, the memory is visceral: the large porcelain sinks at the entrance, the smell of chlorohexidine and the sight of infusion pumps stacked and blinking, ventilators beeping, and monitors alarming. Back then I was afraid to even open the incubators, afraid to touch the babies' thin skin, and more than anything afraid a tube would slip loose. Yet despite my fears I knew I had found what I wanted to do. As terrifying as it was, I felt drawn to the gravity of each decision, the rawness of the experiences, and the feeling that each day I could impact someone's life.

Years before, during college, a friend gave me a book written by her father, Dr. James Judge. *The Closest of Strangers* told the stories of nine patients he cared for as a family practice doctor. I devoured the stories and marveled at the intimacy he experienced with his patients, and especially at the way he saw beyond their illnesses and into the entirety of their lives. The book also told the story of how patient care affected him, the way in which he carried his patients' stories with him and how they changed him. It seemed a beautiful notion, to be so invested and involved that the experiences of others would have a personal impact. I dreamed of becoming that kind of doctor and carried the book with me across the country to Duke, where I completed pediatric and neonatology training. During those years I often worked thirty-hour shifts, trudging into the hospital at dawn and often never leaving at night. What I knew then, and what seemed to matter most, was the objective data: get the diagnosis right, prescribe the correct medications, learn how to insert the spinal needle and place the central line. Confronted with the reality of patient care, those seemingly romantic notions of preserving humanity in medicine drowned under the weight of fatigue, stress, and a crushing workload.

But as the years went by, stories accumulated beneath the outer shell of clinical care. They shifted and swayed in my mind, in a slow reawakening of what had drawn me to medicine and of what mattered most. The stories had become part of who I was and of how I saw the world. One night in late summer, several years after training, I sat in the hospital. Through the blinds I could see the dull orange of the parking lot, the light reflecting off the scattered cars, and clouds of insects swarming the lights. Over my desk the thin fluorescent light bulb hummed. Inside me were the spines of stories and I needed to set the words down, as truly and faithfully as I knew how. Perhaps I was thinking of the many books, like Dr. Judge's, lining my shelves, or perhaps it stemmed from a buried desire to bring my own experiences in medicine to words, a way of working through the accumulation of experiences. I took a breath, my fingers hovered over the keys and sputtered and lurched into the night in question. The world closed in; the night emerged from the fog. The words unraveled.

These are the stories often hidden from view, hidden behind the closed doors of the hospital, and they are the stories of everyday people thrust into great joys and challenges, into circumstances of life and love and loss. As the incidence of physician burnout soars, the attempt to capture truth and humanity in story can help us to notice, to draw near, to bear witness. Stories can moor us when feelings of despair and guilt and futility crest. It is these stories written down in notebooks, on blogs, stowed away on laptops, contained in the books on the bookshelf, which can help us to navigate the waters.

Training

Chameleon

I parked in a dirt lot adjacent to the baseball field and walked across the damp grass towards the hospital. The trees were ragged on the horizon, the clouds mammoth and infinite. Volleys of wind blew through the thin cotton of my scrub pants and spheres of water formed on my jacket. Before me soared the monolithic hospital, stark and white against the gray sky. A year ago, I had driven here white-knuckled, my wife gasping with contractions. Her labor was too advanced for an epidural and so I grasped her hand as tiny capillaries in her cheeks burst and our daughter lurched into the world.

After crossing the wet grass, my shoes damp and water creeping up the edges of my scrub pants, I arrived at the side staff entrance. I worked too few moonlighting shifts for my badge to stay authorized and it blinked red on the side door, so I walked around the side to the emergency room entrance. The metal detector faintly hummed in the small waiting room and an elderly lady coughed phlegm. The faint smell of urine and bleach leached from the linoleum. The security guard wordlessly nodded me through, ignoring the beep as my overnight bag set off the alarm. A tepid uneasiness arose. I was in my first months of newborn critical care subspecialty training, working overnight for extra money at a small local hospital. An attending physician supervised me from home, but she was twenty minutes away.

The unease I felt wasn't without reason. I remembered rounding in the NICU several years earlier, during my internship, standing at the back of the group, frantically jotting down orders, and trying to follow the alphabet soup of neonatology jargon. Behind me I heard the back doors swing open and the flight team strode down the main hallway, pushing a yellow transport stretcher. From my place at the back, all I could see was the small gray body of a baby. Our group followed the flight team into a bay where the baby was lifted onto a radiant warmer. I was too far back to hear their words, but the message got relayed back to me.

"The baby's from Rowan County, two weeks old, got gastric feedings through the IV."

Over a swarm of heads, I could see the fellow, Kyle. His voice was calm and controlled as he methodically called out orders. Through a gap I could see bright lights shining on the baby, a roughly taped breathing tube emerging from colorless lips, his body splayed out and his coloring a slate gray.

"That kid's not gonna make it," whispered another resident. And she was right. He died right there in the bay before we could even admit him to the NICU. We found out that in the hospital where the baby was born, the baby's feeding pump had been inadvertently hooked up to the IV. Several days later I heard that the nurse who made the fatal error had committed suicide.

As I entered the hospital on this moonlighting night, I felt isolated and alone and my mind kept drifting to that day. Over the years I had moved through each phase of training, the responsibility and pressure mounting; now it seemed surreal to have been granted passage to this next level. I hoped I was up to the task. It wouldn't take long for me to find out.

Down empty halls, past the closed registration desk, and up three flights lay the neonatal intensive care unit. Dwarfed in size by the university hospital where I was in training, this community NICU could house just sixteen babies and had limited resources. The only other physicians present in the hospital overnight were an emergency room doctor, an obstetrician, and an anesthesiologist. I both thrived on and felt trepidation at the degree of autonomy I had here, an autonomy not experienced at the university hospital where thick layers of hierarchy dominated decision-making.

Moonlighting hours were sandbags against a rising river of plumbing leaks, rotten sideboards, a failing heating system, dead car batteries, and veterinary bills. I will never forget my feelings of frustration and inadequacy when my son turned four and we couldn't afford to buy him a bicycle. My in-laws came to the rescue and offered to buy it for him.

The evening started off uneventfully. After the customary handoff from the day team, I walked through the NICU to check on babies. The delivery pager was quiet, and I spent several hours in the call room working on a research project. The call room was a little larger than a closet—a bed lay against one wall and small desk with a computer against another. Shelves were cut into the wall and contained a hodgepodge of old medical books and an assortment of medical paraphernalia: breathing tubes, spinal needles, tape, and a chest tube. *People* magazines, lotion, a couple of hand towels, and an old lamp without a lightbulb cluttered the rest of the space. Taped above the desk were dozens of clinical protocols, charts, and phone numbers. With the lights out, one could lie back on the bed and gaze upon the night sky, the heavens illuminated from dozens of luminescent plastic stars affixed to the ceiling.

I worked my way through stacks of research articles. There was a knock on the door and a young nurse, her face flushed, told me of a baby boy who was only several minutes old. He had been born vaginally, at full-term, and after the delivery had cried lustily. "Something's not right; he's half blue," she said. I followed her down the empty hallway to labor and delivery, and as we hurried towards the room, I worried about what I would find. Fluorescent lights gleamed off the hard floor and the long hallway stretched out before me, solemn and stark.

I pushed open the overwide door to the delivery room. The air was pungent and earthy; a primal smell of blood and sweat. Mary O'Sullivan sat propped up in bed, the paleness of her face accentuating freckles that bunched thickly over her high cheekbones and swam across her nose. She didn't seem to see me, her eyes fixed across the room on her newborn's body. The baby lay against the far wall under a radiant warmer. Several nurses stood looking down at his little body. The father, Shaun, stood between mother and child, unsure which to attend to.

The baby's body was shiny, his breath quiet, his chest feathering up and down. He furtively opened his eyes against the light and let out a wail. My eyes took in his coloring and I felt the skin prickle on the back on my neck. Vertically down the center of his body ran a line of demarcation, his skin blue on the left, pink on the right. As I examined him, his arms and legs squirmed normally, and his breaths came in small unlabored undulations. With a stethoscope held against his chest, I could hear the sound of air drawing and re-drawing into his lungs, the heart valves softly opening and closing as the blood gushed past.

The name of the condition came to me: Harlequin, named after the theatrical character's checkered costume. I had encountered it in the middle of a textbook but never in practice. Most of the time it was inconsequential and resolved soon after birth; however, in some cases it could represent a more ominous finding, signaling impending critical illness. I glanced around the room and saw eyes looking expectantly at me. With a nonchalance I didn't feel, I said that we would take him over to the nursery to check his oxygen saturations and observe him.

We swaddled him in a unisex pink-and-blue-striped blanket, slid a blue hat over his partially bald head, and placed him on his mother's chest. "Finnegan," his father whispered into his forehead. "Finn."

After what felt like an age to me and probably only seconds to his mother, I lifted him from her arms and into a bassinet, then wheeled him out of their room. Shaun stayed with Mary and Finn traveled alone—he was only fifteen minutes old and in the hands of strangers. The wheels rolled along the linoleum and the lights sputtered outside the operating room door; I could feel the watchful gaze of several nurses at the nursing station as we bumped onto the carpet of the NICU. The heavy double doors swung shut behind us.

In the darkness of the night there was a hushed reverence, the lighting low, voices quiet and subdued. In stark contrast, the admitting radiant warmer was bathed in bright light. The equipment and instruments set up around it gave it the appearance of a miniature operating room. Several nurses were waiting to receive Finn and quickly applied little sticky pads to his chest and an infrared light probe to his chubby wrist. Immediately the monitors flashed, red and alarmed.

To look at his face was to look at perfection: no awkward molding from the birth canal or bruising from the hardness of the mother's pelvis. Finn had full cheeks and soft butter skin, but the two shades of color on his body were now both darker, midnight blue running into rosewood pink. Before my eyes his breathing became labored, his nostrils flaring slightly at the flanges, the chest skin pulled in between the slats of ribs and belly inverting with the breath. His arms were splayed out without tone or movement. The pulse oximetry alarm showed that the saturation of oxygen in his bloodstream was half of what it should be. I blinked and stood motionless for a second, the flash of the monitor reflecting in slow motion off my glasses. Time grew heavy and compressed. There wasn't time to call for the respiratory therapist. I opened a tackle box and pulled out the laryngoscope and breathing tube. The fingers of my right hand scissored his mouth apart while my left hand guided the metal tip past his tongue and into his throat.

The light probed the darkness; folds of pink tissue swam in clear fluid. Thin bubbles migrated across the surface layer. An almost-audible voice spoke to me, reminding me of past difficult airways, reminding me that the attending was twenty minutes away and that this baby would die if I didn't get the tube in quickly. I inhaled and the training took over, the thirty-hour shifts and eighty-hour weeks. Learning to function in high stress on no sleep had taught me to ignore the voice, to disconnect emotions and focus on what had to be done.

The end of the metal continued to slip down his throat and then, as I slowly retracted it, the epiglottis came into view. With the tip of the laryngoscope blade, I lifted the epiglottis and the pink "V" shape of the vocal cords became visible. I fed the breathing tube into his mouth, down his throat, and curved it up and through the vocal cords. Attaching the tube to the ventilation bag, I let out a sigh of relief—he would be fine once his lungs were expanded and filled with oxygen.

I looked expectantly at the monitor, waiting to see the flashing oxygen saturation start to increase. But it didn't. I tried a little more pressure, slightly faster breaths, but still there was no change. Perhaps a lung had collapsed? I placed a light against each side of his chest and it illuminated his thin skin, small concentric circles visible on the chest wall—his lungs were fully inflated. More numbers flashed on the monitors now and his blood pressure barely registered. In the commotion of intubating him we hadn't called the attending physician. I asked someone to page her.

I dialed a number from memory and a fellow, one year ahead of me at the children's hospital, answered the call. She instinctively knew that a phone call from this hospital at night could only mean one thing: a transport was urgently needed. Minutes later, an ambulance pulled out from the children's hospital, turned left onto a street lit in spheres of yellow, and headed towards me.

I wiped the sweat from my forehead and arranged supplies for a central umbilical line. During the first several days of life, before the vessels scar into strings, the umbilical vessels provided the best chance at gaining intravenous access. At the sink, water threaded down my arms, converging at the point of my elbow before tumbling down onto the black leather of my clogs. After draping the baby's abdomen, I swabbed the cord with rust iron betadine and threaded a tie around the base of the umbilical stump. The white-hot light of the radiant warmer bore into the mesh of my surgical cap and the scalpel sliced through the insensate, gelatinous umbilicus, exposing a single floppy vein and two thick-walled arteries. The warmer cast shrill beeps into the room and sweat built under my stretched gloves; the catheters threaded into Finnegan. I pushed a bolus of normal saline and then ordered a blood pressure drip. I steadied myself to update his parents.

Mary was propped up in bed, alert and tense, the blood drained from her face. Shaun sat on a chair beside her and even sitting, he was tall and lanky; behind wire rimmed glasses his eyes were bloodshot. I caught the dislocated image of the three of us in a mirror over the sink—I felt older than I looked. It seemed as though an age had passed since Finn left this room.

"Finn's really sick," I explained. "We don't know why just yet, but he's not getting enough oxygen into his blood. I've placed him on a ventilator and put in central lines that go right in through his belly button. His blood pressure is low, so we've given him fluid and medicine. I've called the transport team from the children's hospital, and they're on the way. Finn is going to need a lot of support, perhaps even support on a heart-lung machine."

Bewilderment flashed in Mary's eyes. The last time I had talked with them, Finn was only going to the nursery for observation. As I looked at Shaun and Mary, I thought of how time can pass without change as people sleepwalk through the days—counting down until the workday ends or the workweek turns to the weekend or the promotion comes—yet in seconds life can become a tumble of dashed dreams.

When I got back to the unit, his blood pressure was still flashing on the screen and his oxygen saturations hadn't budged. I maxed out the blood pressure drip rate and gave another bolus of normal saline, silencing the alarm which, a minute later, resumed its constant chirping. I tried taking him off the ventilator and using a small bag to squeeze the air into his lungs, but nothing helped. I was sure that the blood vessels in his lungs were constricted and that he needed nitric oxide gas to relax them.

Several minutes later, the doors to the NICU clicked open and I could hear heavy footsteps. The transport trio were dressed in flame-retardant jumpsuits, reflective striping down the sides, the hospital insignia marking the back. They lugged in red jump bags—the cavalry had arrived. They swung the yellowed transport incubator into the bay. The stretcher had a plexiglass square incubator strapped to the top with a built-in ventilator housed underneath and a tiered device for IV pumps at the side. At the end of the stretcher several tanks were fastened, one of which had the markings of nitric oxide. Anticipation tightened my chest as the team hooked up the tank and loosened the valve. The gas hissed as it blended into the line and moved into Finn's lungs. Seconds turned to minutes as the numbers on the monitor flashed. I stood at the end of the warmer silently pleading for his oxygen saturation levels to increase and feeling heavyhearted when they did not. The strange weight of an illogical guilt crested over me—hadn't I done all that I could?

After moving his drips over to their pumps and readying the transport ventilator, the trio scooped him up and moved him into the little plastic box. His head hung limp. With a nod they navigated out of the room. Once they were gone, I wandered back over to the bed space with its used syringes, clear plastic wrappers, and tiny gauze pads, the monitor black, the warmer bright and warm, the room still.

With the door to the call room open, I set into the paperwork, the strange quiet of the unit seeping in as if nothing had happened. While I worked, I played the evening back in my mind, examining events from varying angles. From somewhere deep within, the feeling that I was nothing more than an imposter seeped forth—there would be a knock at the door, and they would escort me out. Yet despite my feelings of inadequacy, I also felt a rush of pride at being at this institution, a place I never would have dreamed I would have the opportunity to practice. My eyes rested on a pen with the hospital insignia stamped on it, and I couldn't believe I was now the one taking care of the patient, no longer hanging back behind more senior physicians, behind the "real" doctors. After years of medical school, of being incapable, of needing direction at every turn; after the years of feeling out of place in the hospital and of being in the way, here I was on the other side.

I wished my grandparents could see me—my English grandfather with a cap and tweed sweater, a retired butler and gardener, and my petite grandmother, almost half his size. Both of their sons left for sea in their midteens and my father went on to college and upper-level management. The change from one generation to the next was readily apparent to me even as a teenager. When I visited my grandparents' house we hand-washed dishes at a stainless steel sink, hung the washing on the line, and read books while my grandfather listened to the horse races on the "wireless." I remember an old black-and-white photograph of them, remember his crisp World War II uniform and confident smile. In the musty basement his wooden-handled tools lined the workbench while my dad spent his vacation checking hundreds of work emails on his laptop in the room above. My grandmother shuffled around the house, serving tea, and clearing dishes. She always appeared so small and frail, but even then, I knew she had a quiet inner strength and determination I could never begin to comprehend. She had seen the Battle of Britain from her front doorstep, had embraced her husband when he returned from the war. I heard stories of her riding a tandem bicycle with my grandfather along the English coast. And I remember my grandfather shifting in his reclining chair, moving a little pillow as he tried to ease the pain. Clipped to his belt, he wore an electric device that delivered little shocks meant to disrupt the pain pathways. He told me stories of lying on barbed wire fences while the other soldiers filed over his back. Even as a teenager, the sacrifices of each generation lay before me.

When Finn arrived at the tertiary hospital he was on the verge of collapse. His oxygen saturations had acutely deteriorated during transport and his heart strained to squeeze blood into the constricted vessels of his lungs. He was in a downward spiral as acid built up in his bloodstream. His pulmonary blood vessels continued constricting, the level of oxygen in his bloodstream diminished, and his heart failed. A small army of physicians, respiratory therapists, and nurses assembled at his bedside and a cardiothoracic surgeon slid large-bore catheters into the blood vessels in Finn's neck. A machine gurgled, running his blood through a myriad of plastic tubes, filtering out carbon dioxide, pumping in oxygen, and returning the blood to his body.

Over the next nine days he remained on the machine, sedated and bloated. Each day his heart gained strength and his lungs improved. On the tenth day, the catheters were removed. If he crashed, he would die, his condition deemed irreversible. Perilously he walked the line and with the cannulas gone, his heart beat and blood coursed through the vessels in his lungs. Carbon dioxide leeched from his bloodstream, expired by his lungs; oxygen diffused into his blood; everything working as it should. Eleven days later, he went home.

No one knows what happened to Finn in the delivery room that night. Doctors discussed his case at the bedside and in the hallways. There were theories and they were good, but unprovable, the prevailing one being that a tiny air bubble made its way from a blood vessel in the placenta into his circulation, causing cardiorespiratory collapse. I still wonder what really happened that night and know that like so many things in medicine, it will probably remain a mystery as elusive as the Loch Ness monster I dreamed of hunting as a child.

Two years passed and I found myself in a room across the hallway from where Finn was born, standing over the warmer of another baby just minutes old. He didn't breathe and his heart rate was slow, stunned by the trauma of eviction. I stood at the head of the warmer, squeezing air into his lungs. I glanced at his mother, her face damp with sweat, hair matted across her brow. A chair was pulled up close to the bed and in it sat Mary O'Sullivan.

Soon the baby wailed, and we placed him on his mother's chest. I turned to Mary with a questioning look and she explained, "I'm here for my friend." It all seemed out of place—Mary tanned, her cheeks full and hair brushed straight, sitting not as a patient but as a visitor. That night years before seemed like a convoluted dream. Now she sat, holding her friend's hand, looking up at me with a knowing smile.

"How's Finn?" I asked.

"Brilliant," she said. "He's brilliant."

What I felt then, and still do to this day, when everything lines up just right and goes according to plan, is a deep gratefulness, a gratefulness borne from experiences when everything crumbles. Below the superficial layers of my own pride is an intuitive humility, an understanding that in every situation we do all we can, but we never ultimately determine the outcome. Finn tested me at a time when I needed to prove myself, to show my ability to work under pressure and to see firsthand the lengths to which technology can go to keep someone alive. He also taught me about hope: that even when it looks as though all is lost, everything can change in unexpected ways.

The Sniper's Son

I carried the confidence Finn had given me through those first months of training, through that time when everything still felt new—placing a breathing tube, putting in an umbilical line, admitting a sick baby. Even the things I had done many times still held the luster of accomplishment. I could measure my growth by looking back over days or weeks. I worked so much that even in my dreams I heard the beeping of alarm monitors, sifted through management decisions from the day, and on more fitful nights, coded babies. A recurring dream was that of a baby crying. In the amorphous way of dreams, it would start out as a baby in the NICU, but when I went to investigate, I would find a baby with a breathing tube in place, the ventilator bellowing air, and yet the crying would continue. Soon I would slip from sleep as my wife rolled out of bed and padded down the hall to feed our daughter. Then I would crash back into dreaming until the morning alarm jolted me from sleep and I would brew coffee and pull the front door closed softly behind me.

Driving to work, the roads were dark and empty, the woods black and foreign. The hospital would emerge, the lighted lettering along the front oval casting shadows. Nurses and doctors shuffled through the pedestrian tunnel, filling the elevators, each floor taking them to entirely different worlds. I exited on the fifth floor, where days melded into nights in the windowless neonatal intensive care unit; every few days I stayed in the hospital for thirty hours until I felt as though I had two homes.

Those months had the infatuation, obsession, intensity, and newness of a honeymoon, and like a young groom I held an unwavering faith—faith in the miracles of modern medicine and deeper still, my belief in a good God. It wasn't that I hadn't experienced heart-wrenching situations before.

Instead, I was just early enough in my training that I still carried the confidence in my own power to prop up the walls between my work and my heart. Everything had a compartment, and in my waking hours I worked hard to keep everything where it belonged. I thought I had learned how to never let on that something affected me, to go home each night and talk with my wife about our children, her day, the house, anything but what went on at the hospital. I thought that my silence starved the emotions. That is why I never told her about the sniper's son.

Three months after my night with Finn, I walked through the NICU in the early afternoon, checking in on babies and nurses. In Pod 4, closest to the hallway I saw a father standing beside an incubator. His hair was cropped short at the sides, flat on top, and he wore combat boots laced over cargo pants. I hadn't seen him before but I knew the mother, who maintained a regular presence by the bedside. I hesitated in the doorway as he stood with his hands on the edge of the incubator, his eyes gazing down through the plexiglass. Surely this was his first time seeing his son. I didn't want to break the moment, and then the monitor beeped and he looked up. When I shook his hand, I could see splotches of acne on his cheeks and patchy teenage stubble.

"Are you in the army?"

"Yes sir, 82nd Airborne—sniper."

He glanced at the monitor, back to the tiny two-week-old baby.

"Well, nice to meet you. I'm Dr. Rattray. I'm taking care of your son. Is this your first time seeing him?"

"Yes—I haven't been able to get up here yet. We just spent a few weeks away on a training exercise." He looked back at his son. "He's so small, I'm afraid to even touch him."

"He's small but he's doing well. We were able to take him off the ventilator a few days ago and he's doing well with his tube feeds. Don't worry about touching him—you won't hurt him."

I opened the side ports of the incubator for him to reach his hands in and the baby's hand folded around the sniper's finger. The father's hand rested on the edge of the mattress, the hand the same thickness and mass as his son's torso. We stood there for a minute in silence until his wife returned from pumping her breast milk, a small clear container in her hand, the yellow fat separating out. She seemed small and girlish next to the sniper, the kind of girl you would see at a high school football game. At ease with her son, she reached in to reposition his head on the blanket and tucked down one arm so that he couldn't pull at his feeding tube. The father stood vigil, unmoving, with the little hand clasped around his finger.

Several days passed, each frantic with new admissions, deliveries, and transports. I walked into work one morning and the overnight physician had an X-ray pulled up on the computer.

"Bad night?"

"Terrible. We got a transport in from Central, three other admissions, and then this," he said, pointing to the film.

I looked over his shoulder and could see the thin slips of ribs; white ground-glass opacities of premature lungs; and a big, full abdomen spilling out under the ribs. The intestines were distended and stacked. Fine lines of black air tracked between the bowel wall layers and up into the liver. The film showed all the hallmark findings of necrotic bowel, a critical disease marked by bacterial overgrowth and, in the end stages, death of the intestinal tissue.

I glanced at the name plate on the film and dread crested over me—it was the sniper's son.

As we prepped him for surgery his blood pressure fell, and the belly grew darker. By mid-morning I sat at the head of the bed and squeezed a synthetic opioid into tubing that tunneled under a blue sterile field into a peripheral vein. Then I chased the opioid with a paralytic to keep his body still during surgery. The surgeon stood over the baby, waiting for the heart to swash the medications through the vessels before starting. Before the surgery, she and I had sat in the little conference room, explaining the procedure and risks to the parents. As usual, she seemed eternally fatigued, prematurely graying, and straightforward. After that a heaviness took up residence and we both fled the room.

As the surgeon ran her scalpel over the abdomen the baby's heart rate rose by twenty beats per minute, and I pushed more opioid into the IV. The surgical spotlight transformed the colors and the dull, bruised abdomen became a roiling blackened sea. After the first strokes of dissection a sheening, glistening wetness emerged, the light dancing like sunlight. More strokes of the blade and the intestines were visible, the violet hue of eggplant. The surgeon ran the loops out over her fingers, every centimeter as dark as the other. As the minutes ticked by, an enveloping knowing settled in, displacing any hope that I had clung to. When she reached the end, our eyes met. She shook her head, scooped the bowel back into the cavity and wordlessly ran sutures across the gaping cavity. I thought of his parents, still sitting in the little conference room, still wondering what the odds were. I thought of what was to come, having to sit next to the surgeon, describing the dead bowel.

I knew we could keep him alive. The respirator could breathe for him, blood pressure medication could keep his blood flowing, antibiotics could cover bacterial translocation from gut to bloodstream, blood and platelet transfusions could keep his numbers in check, and IV nutrition could deliver micro- and macronutrients to his still-functioning liver. I wanted to cling to that hope—just keep him alive and see what happened. We could keep him alive for hours, probably even days, but without intestines he couldn't live a life. I know the surgeon felt the same way because after she closed the abdomen with fine, tight sutures, we talked about offering an intestinal transplant. But the thought was irrational, and we knew it. He was too young and sick. To look at him on the radiant warmer, his body pink and skin soft, a red line cleaved horizontally across his ashen abdomen, and to know that he was alive and would be until we pulled out the breathing tube and IV, caused a hard sinking in my chest. My breaths came out shallow and quick.

Just twenty-four hours ago I had updated his mother—he was doing well, had gained weight. Now there was nothing we could do but let him die in her arms.

Hours later we carried him into a private room, the respiratory therapist hand-bagging breaths into the breathing tube, a wall of IV pumps rolling behind, and placed him in his mother's lap. The sniper sat next to her wearing a formal Army uniform. Five men stood behind the couple, one resting his hand on the sniper's shoulder. My eyes followed the line of men with their lopsided berets, midnight-blue jackets, colored ribbons hanging from their chests, and slacks tucked into jump boots. I looked down at the sniper's baby, the belly black, skin gray, and we slipped the breathing tube from his mouth. The men stood stock-still. I saw the light refract from one man's eyes and watched a tear track down his cheek.

I stood across from them feeling alone in the face of their solidarity. I thought of my wife and I, with our families hundreds of miles away, of how I barely had a friend nearby. I looked at the line of men and then at the young mother and wondered what kind of support she would have once they got home and her husband went back into the field on training exercises; imagined her sitting on the couch in Army housing. I looked up at the men and yearned for that level of belonging—for that deep sense of purpose, to be more than I was. Instead, I stood in my wrinkled scrubs feeling alone and inadequate, selfish, and drained.

I thought about the ways in which we were similar: I, too, worked countless hours, pushed my body past its natural limits, felt the sickening nausea of sleep deprivation. I, too, trained in a hierarchical system and worked for the betterment of other people. Yet I knew that we shared little. The sniper was willing to put his life on the line in ways I couldn't fathom, to hike behind enemy lines, risk capture, torture. My separation from my family only ever lasted thirty hours while his lasted days to weeks. At the end of my training my hours would improve and my pay would increase, while little would change for him—still the wet and the cold and the heavy pack. I knew that it was these truths which separated us and which afforded him a band of brothers. I would remain alone, looking in from the outside, subconsciously drawn towards someone who would make a real sacrifice. I stood there looking at him as his baby slipped away and I couldn't do anything to help.

In the early evening I rode the elevator to the ground floor and used up my cafeteria allowance on sushi, potato chips, and a cold green tea. I took the long way to the parking lot, past the research labs and through a little garden. It was oppressively humid, the air thick, but I breathed it in, grateful to be outside. As I walked, I thought about the upcoming Monday conference. I knew that we would talk about the sniper's baby. We would talk about the risk factors for necrotizing enterocolitis, the type and quantity of the feedings, the feeding progression rate, the choice of antimicrobial coverage, antifungal coverage, the initial radiographs. What we would not talk about would be the sniper, his wife, those men. What we would not talk about would be my feelings of inadequacy. What fumbled words did I say to the parents? How sorry I was; how sorry we were? In the conference I would keep to myself how that evening, as I walked along the winding path, I had wished I could go back in time to my honeymoon in Fiji—to stand on the porch of that little bure, looking out across the lawn with the sound of the waves collapsing on the shore and the songbirds in the trees. How I wished I could slip a kayak through the mangroves again, emerging on an isolated sandy beach. I yearned for that place of freedom. I yearned for my heart that existed then.

I asked a question I would never find the answer to and would never stop asking: why one baby and not the other? Why could we save Finn and not the sniper's son? Why one miracle and not the other?

Even after all these years, I'm still asking the same question, laying down these sentences and sifting through the memories. And when I wonder why I still cling to the story of the sniper's son I remember the words of Ford Madox Ford: "You may well ask why I write. And yet my reasons are quite many. For it is not unusual in human beings who have witnessed the sack of a city or the falling to pieces of a people to desire to set down what they have witnessed for the benefit of the unknown heirs or of generations infinitely remote; or, if you please, just to get the sight out of their heads."

Life forms fissures in our hearts, lines that thread down, divide and track deep underneath. And rebuilding occurs. I yearn for that time in Fiji, but now my marriage is deeper and stronger than before, my heart expands when my daughters smile and say Daddy, when my son walks next to me, his head now level with my clavicles. At times I wonder how I will have the perseverance to do this over the years, to not let myself become crushed under the weight of grief, or worse, to close myself off and feel nothing at all. I wonder if it's normal that I still remember that room, that afternoon, all these years later. I should remember all the babies discharged home with their parents. I should remember them wheeling down the hall and out into the open sunlight, but some stories slip away while others will stay with me forever. I know that this is what I was made to do and that there will be times of action and times of sitting with parents in the unknowing and the pain. I will forget much, so let me write these words and remember the sniper's son.

The Exchange

E very morning during my subspecialty training we rounded as two
separate teams, each covering half of the beds in the intensive care
unit. We started at 8 a.m. sharp and went from pod to pod until just before
lunch. Each team consisted of the attending neonatologist, the fellow, several residents, a pharmacist, nutritionist, the charge nurse, and the bedside nurse. As a second-year fellow I rounded with the nurse practitioner
team while Jeffrey, a new first-year fellow, was assigned to the resident
team. Jeffrey was serious. He wore tortoiseshell glasses and penny loafers.
He had such a strong sense of where he wanted to go in life, such ambi-
tion, that it left me feeling as if I was adrift or had set my sights too low. In
one short year, he had already amassed grant funding and projected the
air of someone far farther along the track than he in fact was.

It was probably for those reasons that the idea struck me. I had noticed
on more than one occasion that Jeffrey kept a stack of blank forms on a
clipboard he carried around for the attending, so that if he ran out of sheets,
Jeffrey could jump in and hand him a fresh one. Late one night as I dragged
myself into the closet of the call room, I noticed the hot pink cover of a
Cosmopolitan shoved in between medical journals. Suddenly, I knew what
I had to do. That night I cut off the front cover, just narrower than a regular
piece of paper, and slipped it under two of Jeffrey's blank rounding sheets.

After rounds the next morning, I asked the residents how it had gone
and got the usual answers: "fine," or "long." The next day, with trepidation
and excitement, I asked the same question, only to get the same answer. It
wasn't until several days later when I was sitting in the computer alcove,
that I overheard the residents talking excitedly, "You should have seen it.
Jeffrey went for a new rounding sheet and there was a *Cosmo* magazine

under it. He started stammering about how it wasn't his." Amidst the stress and long hours, humor helped buoy us up and kept us going.

On the weekends there was only one fellow and an attending who covered the entire unit. That next Saturday, late in the afternoon, we admitted a twelve-hour-old baby boy. His pediatrician called me and, in the background, I could hear a child's laughter interrupted by the playful bark of a dog. A breeze sifted through the trees outside the window, the sun enveloping the shimmering earth, and I thought of children running through the sprinklers, hurling bodies onto the suds of a Slip 'N Slide, the sky a million shades of blue.

The massive air conditioners lumbered out by the back alley. While I gazed out the window, Dr. Clark laid out the story: the hours of life, the blood types of baby and mother, and his last bilirubin level. The number was so high I didn't even have to check the guidelines to know he needed to be admitted. Just ten minutes later, his nurse wheeled him from his mother's room into Room 5, where he lay under a radiant warmer, blond with dimpled cheeks and gray-blue eyes, his skin a buttery yellow. A nurse inserted an IV into the back of his hand and we stripped him naked except for the sliver of a diaper and bathed his body in brilliant blue light. Foam eyeshades wrapped over his eyes; I imagined the blue waveforms permeating his skin, his blood, the jaundice subsiding. His nurse made a cardboard sign with his name in blue letters and attached it to the foot of the bed: "Evan."

Evan's parents came up soon after the admission; his mother, Shelly, sat in a wheelchair, holding his hand and squinting in the effusive light while his father stood behind her, gripping the handles. I introduced myself and explained hyperbilirubinemia, or yellow jaundice. I described how Evan's blood type was different from his mother's, how while he was in the womb the placenta allowed tiny amounts of his blood to mix with his mother's and how her body responded by making antibodies towards this "foreign" blood, antibodies that could cross the placenta into his bloodstream and were programmed to destroy his red blood cells. His mother looked at me quizzically, so I pulled a paper towel from the sink and drew out a picture of a red blood cell and Y-shaped antibodies, some floating freely, others bound to the cell. I went on to show the cell breaking apart, releasing its contents, spilling bilirubin out into the bloodstream. Next, I explained the role of the liver in modifying that bilirubin so the body could excrete it. I told them how babies' livers are immature and slow in processing bilirubin, which allows it to build up in the blood. I described how at high enough levels, the bilirubin can cross the blood-brain barrier and deposit in the brain like tobacco stains on a smoker's fingers, leading to irreversible brain injury. The blue lights change the form of the bilirubin molecule, the waveforms melding into the molecules, silently unhinging them, allowing them to be excreted in the urine and stool. His mother leaned closer to him when I mentioned brain injury and I assured her that we almost never see that now—we have other ways of getting rid of the bilirubin.

What I didn't talk about then was those other ways. It was too soon to go into details which would terrify them, especially when such an event occurred so rarely. In almost every case we start intravenous fluids and phototherapy, and the bilirubin level falls. If that doesn't work or if the level is high to begin with, we give intravenous immune globulin (IVIG) medicine. But it was the most extreme treatment, the treatment of last resort, which I didn't want to go into yet: an exchange transfusion procedure that involved slowly removing twice a baby's blood volume while replacing it with fresh donor blood. That would be a conversation for later if the other measures didn't work.

Kernicterus is Greek for "stained kernel," referring to the way bilirubin preferentially stains the deep core nuclei of the brain. It is so rare that I have never seen a child with it yet I lose sleep over it with a fear so visceral it feels like a weight sliding down my throat and dropping heavily into my stomach. I think of the video clips I have seen of children with kernicterus, the interviews with them and their parents. In one video a teenage boy sits in a wheelchair, his body writhing uncontrollably. He can barely get the sentences out as his head jerks to the side, his jaw twists, and his arms contract. The brain damage preserves one's intellect but ravages the part of the brain that controls movement, leaving a cruelly unwieldy body. One of the most difficult things about the disease is that there is no set bilirubin level at which brain injury occurs in a particular patient. More than half a dozen factors play a role in determining risk: gestational age, blood type incompatibility between mother and baby, hours of age, and clinical illness. Doctors use established guidelines and a nomogram, a special graph that factors in these variables, to plot a baby's age and bilirubin level to determine the type of treatment that should be offered. The nomogram, however, is limited to babies over thirty-five weeks gestational age, leaving us to make educated conjectures about premature infants. There are some things in life that are cut-and-dried and most of us build our lives around such certainties. Yet most of medicine lives in the shadowland of grays, in the weighing of costs and benefits without the luxury of complete information. If we follow the nomograms, it is unlikely that a baby will get kernicterus, but there are a myriad of factors that can modulate the outcome and more questions than answers: does it matter how long the bilirubin level is above the treatment threshold or how far above the level it is until the molecules begin to deposit? How does the blood protein concentration and rate of rise affect risk? Are some babies more genetically vulnerable?

The next bilirubin check was scheduled four hours after admission to give the fluids and phototherapy time to work. With a faith born of experience and bolstered by optimism, I expected the level to drop. Yet the next level had risen by several points, a steady climb slowed but not stopped by our efforts. I sighed and graphed the level on the nomogram. We were getting close to the exchange transfusion threshold, that unyielding black line on the page. I took the stairs down to his parents' room, walking under a burden of worry, praying that we would be able to get the level turned around.

His parents were watching TV and I sat on the vinyl-lined couch by the window and told them the results. I explained that we would need to give IVIG and had them sign a form releasing us to give the blood product. This time I told them about exchange transfusions, the process of inserting central lines, removing small quantities of blood, and exchanging it for fresh blood. Worry creased Shelly's face and I quickly assured her that we almost never have to perform an exchange transfusion, that we hadn't done one in this hospital for several years. What I didn't tell them about were my own concerns: that I had only done the procedure once before, several years prior, and that I hoped we had all the right supplies, that the nurses knew how to set up the blood warmer and that the blood bank would be able to quickly send us the type of blood we needed. I didn't confess that I hoped that I could remember the nuances of how to set up the tubing and the stopcocks, nor did I reveal my irrational fear of losing track of how much blood we had taken and given, of getting the numbers mixed up and either taking too much or giving back too little. My older colleagues tell stories of performing two exchange transfusions in one night, ten in a week, but now with more effective treatments—modern phototherapy, medicine to prevent immune reactions—the younger generation might go through their entire training without having to do even one. In fact, I was lucky to have the experience of performing one already. And still the prospect of performing an exchange made me uneasy, the thought of removing twice a baby's blood volume and replacing it with someone else's blood; the fluid shifts, electrolyte imbalances, risk of cardiac arrythmia; the need for meticulous counting of the milliliters out and in and the need for the new blood to be prepared to the right concentration of red blood cells, the potassium content low enough, then warmed to the right temperature. I smiled at them with a plastered-on confidence and reassured them that the immunoglobulin would work, then walked back down the hall wishing I could be unmoored from this.

Back in the office, as I ordered IVIG and a repeat bilirubin level for two hours later, my phone rang. It was a nurse from the mother/baby floor who sounded tired and apologetic. She was caring for a mother who had a baby in the NICU. The mother was upset and said that she hadn't been updated that day and needed someone to come and speak with her. By that time, it was almost seven and I wanted to eat my dinner and call home as I always did on call nights to say goodnight to my kids before they went to bed. I quickly called home, feeling rushed, not wanting to keep the mother waiting, and then headed to her room. I had already met her that morning at the bedside after rounds and we had talked about her daughter's condition and our current treatment plan. Prior to delivery her baby had a bowel movement in the womb, the brown particulate matter bathing her vernix-covered skin, and when she took her first breath the particles drew into her lungs, physically obstructing the tiny terminal air sacs and chemically inflaming the tissue. She lay on a bed in the NICU on a ventilator, needing 50 percent oxygen and high ventilatory pressures. She had central umbilical lines in place and was on intravenous nutrition and antibiotics. As I walked towards the room I thought of the father, of how I had walked him up from the delivery room, his frame thin and wiry, his cheeks sunken and hollow, teeth rotted out, eyes blue. He said little. Before my knuckles struck the door to knock, I could hear a woman's raised voice. I could only pick out a few words, mostly expletives, and she was either on the phone or talking to herself. My stomach grumbled and I thought of the dinner that I had put in the microwave just before the nurse called me. When I entered the room, the mother was alone, pacing along the side of the bed. She hunched over a little at the waist, one hand on the small of her back, her straight brown hair hanging over her freckled cheeks. Her eyes narrowed when they fixed on me.

"The doctor last night told me she could go home tomorrow. He said that you would take her off the ventilator today. I can't take this shit. My husband has to get back to work and I have to take care of my other kids."

I took a breath, trying to achieve a firm but understanding tone. "Harmony is really sick right now. The ventilator is working hard, and we are having to give her quite a lot of oxygen."

"Well, you need to discharge her so we can get home," she repeated. "I've got other kids at home—I'll take her to appointments. I want to do this outpatient."

I blinked, looked at the clock and steadied my breath. "Look, we want the same thing as you. We would love for her to go home. As soon as we can get her off the ventilator, get the central lines out and have her feeding by herself, she'll be ready to go home with you."

Her eyes flared, "I read an article that the NICU causes the problems it's supposed to treat. When I go up there no one tells me anything. They told me they have to help me get her out of the bed to hold her. She's my daughter, I know how to hold her. They don't need to treat me like I don't know what I'm doing. Anyway, she does fine when I'm there—she just needs to be home with me."

My eyes felt like sandpaper and a righteous indignation crested over me. I had bigger things to worry about than pacifying an unappreciative, angry mother. I might have to do an exchange transfusion in a few hours, this mother's baby was horribly sick, and we had another baby whose breathing was becoming erratic. I thought of the long night ahead of me and allowed myself to wallow in self-pity. I thought of people with eight-to-five desk jobs, of my neighbor in finance and another who owns his own company. Did they have to deal with crazy people who can't be reasoned with? Did they feel the heaped-on pressure like bricks on their backs and tightness in their chests? I thought of a few calculated words to let her know how irrational she was being and then as I drew in a breath, saw her bare feet and, in her hard eyes, a mother's love—fiercely defensive and wild. Suddenly, I stood chastened, feeling ungrateful and entitled. Who was I to judge the roiling emotions of a mother with a sick baby and other children to care for at home? I, who stood in front of her with the greatest privilege society can give to a person: the unparalleled privilege to care for the sick. I get to do what I love, what I feel called to do. While millions of people work under abusive bosses in jobs that barely pay enough, in jobs they hate, I have the blessing of working with my hands and mind to care for babies.

"It's wonderful that you want to hold her. You know, it can be really beneficial for babies to be held. We don't mean to offend you by helping you with getting her out of the bed, it's just that if the central line comes loose, she could bleed and lose a lot of blood and if the breathing tube comes out her oxygen saturations would go really low. We just want to keep her safe. I know this is hard but we're going to do everything we can to get her better and home to you as soon as possible—just bear with us for a little longer."

"What happens if I want to take her home? You can't stop me."

The conversation had gone on long enough and was veering towards a confrontation that I didn't want to get into. "I'm sorry, but we can't allow you to take her home right now. She would die if we took her off the ventilator."

"You don't know that; you don't know that she would die."

"Well, we are about 99.9 percent sure she would die, she's really sick right now."

She persisted, "Well, you can't stop me. There's nothing you can do to stop me."

I tried to stop my blood pressure from rising, to keep my voice calm. I looked at her flatly. "If you try to take her, we will have to call security."

She looked at me hard, got a little closer to me and mustered up all the malice she could in her voice. "I'm going to call the DEA," she threatened, then stood back like she had just won a debate.

"The Drug Enforcement Agency? Feel free to call anyone you want." I squirted cold alcohol foam on my hands, pulled open the door, and stepped into the hallway. I could hear her cursing me as the door clicked shut.

Later that evening I checked on Evan, his breaths coming in small sighs, the blue lights spotlighting him, their intensity darkening the periphery of the room. The immunoglobulin bag hung empty on the pole. There was no way of knowing his bilirubin level by looking at him. In the past, trainees were taught to look at the watermark to which the yellow jaundice tracked up—the nipples, neck, over the face—to estimate the bilirubin load, but we know now that such estimates are completely inaccurate. A few minutes later I watched while a lab tech lanced Evan's heel and dripped blood into a small green container. Each bluish drop slid down the side of the plastic until it reached the full line on the side of the tube. I thought about that vial of Evan's blood going to the lab and running through the machine, of the results that would determine the trajectory of the night and perhaps even Evan's life like the volatile path of a tornado that can turn on a dime, leaving one house unscathed while it levels the house next door.

I went across the hallway to the office and impatiently tapped through emails from the day. My inbox was cluttered with duplicate hospital announcements, one from the executive sending it and the same email forwarded from the secretary. There were fifteen emails marked critical from the IT department about outages for systems that I didn't know existed. I deleted the messages without reading them and kept checking the medical record for the lab to come back, but after forty-five minutes the box was still blank, and I called down to the lab. After giving the medical record number, verifying the last name, and waiting on hold the tech came back on the line and informed me that we hadn't collected enough blood—the machine couldn't read the sample.

"I saw them fill it to the line," I protested angrily. I could hear the wiring of machinery in the background; she blandly told me it couldn't run. I switched to pleading.

"We need to know what to do right now—it's an emergency, the last level was rising. He's a baby."

"Do you want to send another one?"

I rubbed my eyes, "Yes, we'll send a new one, can you run it right away?"

When I went in to tell Evan's nurse about the lab problem, I walked past Harmony's room. Her nurse flagged me down to tell me that her mother had just visited and managed to pull her out of the bed when the nurse's back was turned. As she pulled Harmony out, the endotracheal tube had been pushed deep, setting off ventilator alarms, and the central line had snagged on the edge of the warmer, stretching it, but the suture had held the line in place. They now were having to watch the mother constantly, ready to jump in anytime she made a move. I told them if it happened again, we would have to call security—there was too much risk to the baby.

I found Evan's parents at the bedside anxiously awaiting the lab results. Apologetically, I explained the problem and reassured them we would run a new sample immediately.

"They couldn't run the sample?" asked his father, leaning forward in his chair, the pitch of his voice rising.

Like a used-car salesman, I stood there apologizing, trying to keep a clear head when I knew it wasn't fair or right or just. I spitefully wished that it wasn't me who was tasked with telling parents about the lab problems. I wondered how the administrators who had decided to outsource the lab as a cost-cutting measure would feel standing there in front of Evan's parents, a little before midnight, the neurotoxin building in his bloodstream.

An hour and twenty minutes later the nurse called with the bilirubin level and my heart sank. It had continued to rise steadily, and we were now into the exchange transfusion zone. I logged into the computer to double-check, then refreshed the screen and checked the time stamp on the lab, then rechecked it against the nomogram. I couldn't believe the IVIG hadn't worked.

I called the attending at home to tell him the results and my plan for an exchange transfusion. "Okay, call me if you need me; need me if you call me," he said. It may sound like a flippant response, but his statement communicated both his trust in me and his support—I knew he would be there in minutes any time of the day or night if I needed him.

I walked briskly to the parents' room where I found them asleep, the mother in the hospital bed and the father on a fold-out cot. It struck me how strange it is that parents sleep in separate beds in the hospital. Couples may not have slept apart for years and yet here in the hospital with all the stress and sickness, they are separated. My fingers accidently landed on the main overhead light instead of the softer one over the sink. Shelly woke immediately and in the bright light she had hopeful eyes and rounded cheeks. She reached over and shook her husband awake and I felt awkward as he rolled over, shirtless, and rubbed his eyes, propping himself up on one elbow.

I pulled up a chair and watched Shelly's face fall as she realized why I was there. I had so much to say and the clock was ticking. Evan's bilirubin level was rising as I walked down the hallway to their room, while I sat on the chair and spoke, while we called the blood bank and prepared for the transfusion. I thought about how I wished I had gone into every detail of an exchange transfusion earlier in the day, but at that time it had seemed so unlikely. I began telling them about Evan's increased bilirubin level and the need for an immediate exchange transfusion; the need to put in central lines, pull off small quantities of blood, and replace it with fresh blood until we had replaced twice his blood volume.

His mother looked at me, unbelieving. "You're going to take out all of his blood twice and replace it?" It wasn't really a question, more of a repetition of something outlandish.

"Yes, but we'll do it slowly, over hours, little bits at a time—it's the only way to get rid of enough bilirubin. We rarely do this procedure and it's usually well tolerated; however, I should warn you that as with any procedure there can be complications."

"What kind of complications?" his father interjected.

I ran through the risks related to central line placement: risks from the blood itself; the extremely low risks of infections such as HIV, hepatitis B or C carried by the blood; then risks related to fluid shifts and electrolyte shifts.

"We're going to take good care of Evan. I'll update you when we're finished," I assured them and hastily left the room.

It was late, almost one in the morning, and I made my way back to the office, my mind spinning with logistics, amped up on adrenaline. The night stretched before me, seven hours until relief would come. I caught my reflection in the black window, the light bright on the height of my forehead; the smell of burnt coffee plunging me back to my previous sleepless nights of training. Nights of loneliness and breakpoint exhaustion supported by a current of adrenaline.

In the office, I pulled a blank sheet of paper off the printer and wrote out the equation for the amount of blood to transfuse, 120 milliliters of blood times his weight in kilograms times two, plus 40 milliliters for the dead space in the tubing, then pulled a stout book off the shelf and rechecked my work. It was quiet, like the whole world was asleep while our drama played out here on our isolated little island. I called the blood bank and a technician with a southern drawl answered. I talked through the order: typed and cross-matched fresh blood, reconstituted to a hematocrit of 45, to be sent Stat to the NICU.

When I went to his bedside it was already getting crowded with equipment—the blood warmer, a cart with an array of syringes and supplies—and the area was cordoned off with folding screens. While the nurses bustled about, I scrubbed up and worked on placing umbilical venous and arterial central lines. I had to work with the blue bilirubin lights off so that I could see the vessels and I moved as quickly as possible to minimize the time the lights were off. In some ways it didn't really matter, as we would be removing twice his volume of blood and replacing it with fresh blood, but in the meantime, I wanted him to get all the phototherapy possible. The umbilical line stopped short several times, bouncing off the spongy liver, and I couldn't draw blood back. But then I tried again with a little spin of the line and inward pressure on the liver and the line went freely, on up through the ductus venosus towards the right atrium of the heart. I dilated one of the thick-walled spirals of the umbilical artery and pushed the tip of the catheter down into it until it gave, and a line of red threaded up through the catheter.

The room grew busier as I finished securing the lines. Under the bright lights, several nurses hung a bag of blood on an IV pole and attached tubing that fed into the warming machine. We worked together to attach two three-way valves in tandem so fresh blood could be drawn into the tubing and pushed with a syringe into the umbilical line, then the stops turned so that by pulling back on the stopper, blood could be pulled from the baby, the stopper turned, and the blood squirted into a waste bag.

Once everything was set, I sat down to start the tedious process of removing and replacing ten milliliters of blood at a time. After each tiny transfusion the bedside nurse jotted down the numbers. Each ten-milliliter removal or replacement had to happen slowly over a two-to-three-minute span so that there wouldn't be significant fluid shifts. I could feel beads of sweat tracking down my forehead, pooling along my eyebrows, and my glasses kept slipping down the bridge of my nose. I watched the bedside monitor for arrythmia and kept my own silent tally of our progress, calculating that the procedure should take about an hour and a half to two hours if I maintained the correct, steady pace. Sitting on the stool with the long, drawn-out minutes, there was little else to do but think and worry. Mostly, I worried about his calcium level dropping and setting off an arrythmia and I worried about whether we were dropping his bilirubin level fast enough. I thought back to a story an attending had told me about losing a baby to an arrythmia—they had injected calcium and given epinephrine, but before they knew what had happened, he was gone.

If I could peer into the white matter of Evan's brain and see the bilirubin molecules, would I see them washed up on the banks of his basal ganglia, lining the thalamus? I sent a set of electrolytes to the lab and periodically checked the monitor. Every so often I squinted at the tiny waveforms, imagining the peaks and ridges elongating, flattening, before the heart stopped beating. I looked at the syringe of calcium on the chart, then blinked again and realized that the waveform was normal. At one point I could hear his parents' voices on the other side of the screen, asking the nurse how things were going and when we would be finished.

The next time I looked up at the monitor I saw the telltale flattening of the first wave form, the widening of the ventricular beats. It was like looking at an oncoming car and I sat for an instant in disbelief. Bucking the trance, I grabbed a syringe of calcium, injected it faster than I should have, and chased it with a normal saline flush to move the calcium through the tubing into Evan's bloodstream. I sat there barely breathing as his heartbeat wobbled, careened to the side, corrected itself, then leveled off. I breathed a sigh of relief. The smell of old deodorant seeped from under my shirt and my mouth tasted sour and dry. Ten syringes later I smiled at the nurse recording. "We did it, right? All done?"

"Yeah—that was the last one."

I sent another bilirubin level to the lab and went to update his parents. In a way it was anticlimactic; there wasn't much to say, simply that the procedure was over, and we had given calcium to correct a transient arrythmia but that otherwise he had tolerated it well. We would have a new level within the next hour.

It was four thirty in the morning by the time I slumped onto the call room bed. I was too wired and anxious to sleep so I sat and flipped through the TV's channels, finally landing on a movie where a grimy, wiry man chased a man and woman through a deserted barn. I needed something mindless to move the clock until the results came back. I kept thinking of what the number might be. Surely, a 50 percent reduction would be too much to hope for. At that point I would have been happy with anything low enough to get by without having to do another exchange that night. Something low enough for us to get out of the danger zone for brain injury, for the night's worth of effort to be of benefit. I got up every fifteen minutes to check the computer in the office and by five fifteen the new number emerged on the screen. I looked at the number, double-checked the time and date stamp, and slumped back in my seat. It had dropped by eight points and was below the exchange transfusion threshold. Evan was out of danger.

As the sun's first light shone through the blinds, I leaned back in my chair, spent adrenaline seeping from my bloodstream. I realized that moments like these, moments when catastrophe is averted and we stand on the other side unscathed, with the baby sleeping under the radiant warmer, his eyes fluttering under his thin eyelids and his pudgy arms against his sides—these are the moments I will always remember.

Far from Home

During my years in pediatric residency, while walking from the parking lot to the main entrance of the hospital, I would often see a helicopter taking off from the roof, the steady throb of the rotors ricocheting off the buildings. I would watch the bright blue of its belly as it surged away, banking over the undergraduate campus. Slogging into work, the sight of the helicopter lifting always filled me with a sense of excitement—there was action and meaning and immediacy in the way it roared off the roof only to disappear into the horizon. The element of danger added to the effect. I had seen the flight nurses with their stenciled helmets and visors, their flight suits, and heavy black boots. As someone from the *Top Gun* generation, I was moved.

Only a few years later, I would have my turn. As a newborn critical care fellow, I ended up carrying the transport pager 24-7. Anytime the crew needed to get a sick baby, the call would go out and any available fellow was expected to go. As it happened, out of our eight-person group, there were always several people who couldn't go—maternity leave, fear of flying, or exhaustion from having worked the night before. For those reasons I ended up going on transports frequently, and for the most part I didn't mind. They paid me moonlighting pay and it was a unique chance to take care of sick babies in a completely different environment.

I was in my last year of fellowship, year six after medical school. My oldest was now in kindergarten; my two daughters, three years old and six months old, were born during my training. Our beagle was now gray around the eyes and starting to slow down. We slept in a four-bedroom house, white with black shutters and a red door. A gentle breeze enticed a flowering tree to scatter pink petals onto the front steps and an oak reached out its branches and scratched the siding. Outside the front window a fluorescent streetlamp cast a damp yellow haze and the night was quiet. Inside, on a bedside table, my pager came alive, piercing the silence. My wife stirred and turned over. The bedside clock glowed red: 2:10 a.m. I tiptoed into the bathroom, closed the door and, hoping not to wake the children, dialed the neonatal intensive care unit.

The house sighed and shifted, dreams floating through my children's rooms. Elevator music played on the phone line, and a tired nausea crept over me. I opened the bathroom blinds and looked over the backyard. Below me familiar objects lay swathed in pale light: a sandbox, a soccer ball, a thin paved walking path winding past the back gate. I thought of my children toddling, then walking, down that pathway, picking up leaves and sticks, the small stream tumbling along beside us and my wife and I holding hands, giddy with the sheer wonder of it all.

Abruptly, a voice came on the line, curtailing my reverie; there was a sick baby to the east. The helicopter crew was readying the craft. With adrenaline seeping into my bloodstream, I splashed cool water on my face and brushed my teeth. In the dark I felt for a pair of soft, well-worn scrubs. I kissed my groggy wife, warm and comfortable. From the front stoop, I gazed over the sleeping neighborhood; the night was still and soft, and my heartbeat was fast.

The streets were desolate as I drove to the hospital. Wisps of fog crept out from the woods, licking the road. A doe stood half-hidden behind a loblolly pine, eyes unblinking, tawny antlers still as a branch in the streak of the headlights. I wondered how sick the baby was and whether I would be able to get him back to the hospital alive.

Only the first two stories of the large five-deck parking garage were occupied. Beyond the garage lay a college campus lined with oaks and dotted with Gothic-style buildings. At its heart a cathedral reached into the sky. Far above me on the roof, helicopter blades throbbed in the air. I stopped at the back door of the intensive care unit for tiny bags of blood pressure medication, a central line kit, and a chest tube kit. Continuing up the stairs, two at a time, I emerged out of breath on the rooftop helipad.

On the rooftop, the wind gusted up over the ridge of the building, safety nets strung around the periphery, constellations of demarcation lights, webbed steel walkways, the sleeping city unfolding below. The crew had already loaded the empty transport incubator and were finishing up the last checks when I arrived. I stuffed in earplugs, pulled on a helmet, and climbed into the cockpit. The pilot was going through the final checks and barely acknowledged me, his face glowing in the light of hundreds of tiny buttons and switches. Cropped white stubble grew from sun-weathered skin and even in the small cockpit he moved with a purposeful swagger that made me feel small and out of place. "Hot on one, hot on two, visual checks performed, ready for mission with four souls on board."

In an instant the craft rose vertically before plunging off the lighted roofline into the dark. Beneath my feet I watched the old Gothic cathedral slip away. We tracked a beaded string of parallel lights far below until, for a moment, I was suspended fifteen hundred feet above my sleeping wife and children, looking down on my life, before being pulled away as we banked to the east.

Soon we left the city, flying over dark wooded areas and pastures with only occasional roads and lights. Out the domed front window, sparse clouds drifted under the moon. Below us lay a lake, its water still and inky. From the shallows, the lake crept onto the land, black fading into black.

Minutes turned into miles with the droning of the motor, my loneliness and isolation building. Forty-five minutes passed and the line of the horizon imperceptibly became lighter as we peered into the precursor of the dawn.

Soon, miniature yellow lights threaded underneath and the pilot motioned to a three-story building. We crested a tree line and dropped onto a gray square fringed by a chain-link fence. Outside the window, the pulse of the blades flattened the tall grass and gauzy fog seeped over the tarmac. We landed with a slight bump, and as we stepped out onto the concrete the air was heavy and humid, cicadas chirping loudly as John and Ed, the flight nurses, pushed the two-hundred-pound transport incubator down the path to the entrance of the hospital.

We hurried into the building, the pilot nearing the maximum number of hours in a row he could work. We had exactly forty-five minutes to stabilize the baby and get back to the helicopter. Otherwise, we would be stuck waiting for either a ground ambulance or a new craft.

The hospital lobby vaulted up three stories, all glass and wooden beams, new hardwood floors, and silk ficus plants. It was deserted except for a middle-aged couple slumped in leather chairs near the front doors. They looked up at us as we passed, an army of three. We wheeled down a maze of empty halls, past the steady eyes of hospital founders and leaders watching from the walls.

Soon we clicked through the door of the small nursery, our eyes drawn to several people congregated around a warmer bed. Four babies slept peacefully in open cribs around the periphery of the room. The pediatrician, Dr. Anderson, stretched out a lanky arm and gripped my hand. His handshake was warm and eager. A respiratory therapist stood by the bedside squeezing air into the baby's mouth and nose while a jittery nurse stood at the base of the bed attempting to coax a small volume of blood into a lab tube. One of the flight nurses took over bagging air into the baby's lungs while the other set up our transport ventilator. I worked on getting together supplies to place a breathing tube while Dr. Anderson described the events of the evening.

The mother had been admitted the day before, sweating in the heat of the day, sweating in the cool of the hospital bed, abdomen cramping. She was only in her early twenties, but she was already accustomed to this area of the hospital. In her first pregnancy she had delivered a healthy girl; in her next, a stillborn son. He had been five weeks from the due date when she stopped feeling him move.

Now for the third time, perhaps in the same room, she gave birth. Once again, the baby was five weeks early and after the familiar cramping and nausea her body expelled him in a traitorous act of self-preservation. I pictured each detail as Dr. Anderson recounted the story: the room filled with the welcome wail at the injustice of cool air and bright lights. Slippery and smooth, Cash sprawled on his mother's damp chest, blinking furtively in the light, his father's calloused hands resting gently on his back.

For the first twenty minutes he lay like that until his breath quickened, his little nostrils flared, and his soft, pliable chest wall sucked inwards on each breath. The normal newborn bluish hue on his hands and feet crept towards his core, covering his chest and face. Quickly, he was wheeled down the hall to the nursery where an oxygen-filled clear plastic tent covered his head and torso, an IV jutted into his wrist and antibiotics dripped into him.

Cash's oxygen saturations improved in the tent, the oxygen content in his bloodstream increasing, his red blood cells greedily tethering free oxygen molecules to themselves. He squirmed vigorously, so Dr. Anderson left his number with the nurse and went home. It seemed that the squall had passed.

Shortly before two o'clock his phone rang: Cash was blue and struggling to breathe. Dr. Anderson drove with one hand on the wheel, the other holding his cell phone, calling our hospital for help.

As he stood in the little nursery with the pulse oximeter beeping low, the baby's breaths concaving the chest wall and the arms and legs motionless, the wait for the helicopter must have seemed like an eternity. Cash's heart rate spun down every time Dr. Anderson tried to place the breathing tube—each time, instead of curving up and through the small, tight vocal cords, the tube slipped at the last second and took the straight path into the esophagus. His stomach filled with air and the lungs were quiet. Soon they had to stop trying and instead squeezed air from a bag into his mouth and nose.

As I listened to Dr. Anderson's account I looked down at Cash under the bright light of the warmer. The colors told a story: blue-gray skin for low oxygen content; white translucent fingernails for poor circulation; and the sheen of swollen, taut skin as fluid leached from his blood vessels into his tissue.

Dr. Anderson finished speaking and, as if on cue, Cash's heart rate slowed, dropping ten beats each second, until there was just a flat red line on the monitor. John, the flight nurse, pushed his meaty fingers rhythmically down into Cash's chest wall. I guided a breathing tube into the trachea and Ed pulled epinephrine into a syringe. Oxygen and epinephrine molecules bumped and crashed in the tunnels of his bloodstream. Then the heartbeat resonated in his chest, its rhythm ascending the tubes of the stethoscope, and I let out a held breath.

With Cash's heart beating steadily, John and Ed worked on the tangle of monitor lines, IV tubing, and transport ventilator tubing. I scrubbed my hands and set about placing central umbilical lines. A sympathetic nurse came into the room with three cans of Coke and set them by the sink for us. Under the lights of the warmer, with a surgical gown sticking to my sweat and a mask fogging the lower rims of my glasses, I could see the beads of condensation on the cans. My heart thrummed with adrenaline, the umbilical vessels sheening in the light.

I pictured the pilot glancing at his watch, the minutes marching on—there was still a chance of making it to the helicopter in time. While the flight nurses moved Cash into the transport incubator, I hurried down a dim hallway to the parents' room. Knocking softly, the door gave way to gloomy darkness. The air was stale with the smell of tobacco and last night's pizza. In the dark I felt for the light switch and a single tube flickered over the mother's bed.

She slept propped up on two pillows, her face pale and rounded. A hospital gown hung loosely from her neck, clear IV tubing tracked down her left forearm, and a yellow Foley tube emerged from under her gown. To her right, the bulk of Cash's father was crumpled into a half-reclined armchair. He rested tangled in a white hospital sheet, heavy snores rolling off his chest.

Cash's mother woke first, reaching out an arm to shake her husband. I stood over the bed, a stranger. The words came out more quickly than I wanted them to, but the parents nodded and seemed to follow along. I promised that we would wheel Cash into their room before flying out.

I clicked open the door to the nursery and as I entered, the heart rate monitor stabbed the air. Cash lay still, blue creeping over him, and his heart stopped beating. Like a pit crew, we launched into our repertoire, checking the breathing tube, giving epinephrine and fluids. I shined a light onto his chest looking for lung collapse but there was none. On his chest, the metal rim of the stethoscope rested still. Below my fingers, I felt only solidness and coolness.

Sodium bicarbonate to buffer acid. Epinephrine every three minutes. Normal saline boluses every five minutes. Chest compressions and breaths. My mind felt sluggish as I tried to find some connection between the previous stillbirth and this sick baby. I had told the parents we would be by in a few minutes. Time tightened, another revolution of the minute hand. Outside in the approaching dawn, the pilot readied to leave.

Still, Cash's heart did not beat. There was a chance that fluid had accumulated around his heart, compressing and strangling it. With nothing to lose, I painted under the bottom of his left rib cage, brown Betadine swirls bleeding down onto the white linen. Under the rib cage the needle angled towards his heart while I pulled back every so often, but each time the syringe remained empty. Deeper until, surely, I was in the heart—the needle almost out of length and then the give, straw-colored fluid coursing into the syringe up to the 4-milliliter mark as the fluid choking his heart drained. Like an apparition, numbers appeared on the monitor and color swept over him, a sort of pale pink. I slid the needle out.

Ten minutes later, the cold sugary fizz of Coke slipped down my throat and I saw Cash's heart rate nosedive on the monitor from across the room. Everything again. That time only 2 milliliters of fluid flowed back into the syringe, but the heartbeat came back.

Cash's parents were brought into the nursery, the locked door clicking open mechanically. The nurse pushed the mother, engulfed in an oversized wheelchair, IV pole lurching along beside her, face riveted on her son. Two steps behind, disjointed by the gravity of the situation, trudged the father. He seemed out of place in the nursery with his thick work boots and stained jean shirt. He stood with his eyes fixed on his baby, his body moored to the wheelchair.

Cash's mother held his little hand and I described the chain of events, my eyes drawn to the splotch of Betadine under his ribs and the empty syringes, gloves, and piece of blood-spotted gauze littering the floor. They stared at Cash as I spoke, avoiding my eyes, faces unmoving, unflinching. When I told his mother how sorry I was, I put my hand on her shoulder, but it felt contrived and artificial and I pulled it back awkwardly towards me.

They had such little time with him before his heart stopped again. A nurse guided them back from the warmer and this time we worked in front of them. From behind me I could hear the father pleading with us to do everything. I was tired and my heart was heavy. When I sank the needle under the rib once again, there was no return of fluid. I looked at the clock and ended the resuscitation. His father crouched, making guttural sounds, while his mother sat in the wheelchair, her face covered in tears. Another baby lost.

I stood there as an outsider to their grief, wanting to offer comfort yet having nothing to give. I lingered, trying to show our care and sorrow, but it was time for us to leave. The crew needed to get home and sleep. And so we left, the baby lying white on the warmer and the parents hunched over.

It was a strange and empty feeling, walking back down the carpeted hospital hallways as the lobby filled with people. My throat felt tight, my body weary with the loss. We stepped into the sunlight as if moving between dreams and waking.

The helipad was empty. Three hours had passed. An oversized ambulance truck from our hospital had already arrived and was waiting for us in the emergency room bay. We swung open the back doors and threw in the jump bags, clicked the gurney in, collapsing the legs as it slid along the tracks. I hauled myself onto the bench.

Out the window the marshland turned to fields, then suburbia. Morning commuters slipped past us, drinking coffee, cell phones pressed to ears, embarking on a day they would most likely forget.

As I gazed out the window, I felt numb. The image of the father gripping the wheelchair and the mother with her wild hair and tear-stained face kept flashing before me, and I realized that with the passage of time, something within me had eroded. I wanted to go back to who I was prior to medical training; to recover that innocence and optimism; to jettison the weight of responsibility. I wanted to move back into the idealism I felt during a college medical mission trip to Mexico or while working on research with a mentor during medical school, but when I thought back on those times it seemed as if I was looking back at a different person. Sitting on the bench of that ambulance, staring at the empty incubator, I wondered if God was really as good as I had always believed.

By the time I pulled into my driveway the sun was bright and the day warm and lazy. White blossoms on the pear trees and yellow pollen spreading its coat over the surface of the earth. As I walked up the driveway, I could hear the sound of children's giggles. My wife in shorts and a T-shirt, hair pulled back into a ponytail, with our baby on her hip. The baby grinned, all spunk and life with her two little teeth and a rainbow-colored tank top. My three-year-old daughter was a blur of blonde-headed motion as she chased my son around a tree. "Daddy's home!" they called as they ran to me.

It seemed that moving through that side gate should create a transition from my work overnight as a physician to my role at home. But I crossed that threshold drenched in a sense of failure, my mind clouded with the tragedy. Seeing the faces of my wife and children, something swelled within me. Tired and grieving, I moved towards them.

— PART TWO ————————————————————

Young Attending

The Road Home

After three years of pediatric residency training followed by another three years of neonatology fellowship training, I fed my dirty scrubs into the scrub-dispensing machine one last time, turned in my keys, and walked across the road, away from the university hospital. I was thirty-three years old and about to start my new job at a large community neonatal intensive care unit. After ten years of supervision, I was on my own, and while I could call a colleague to discuss something if I needed, the weight of the decisions ultimately rested on me. Perhaps that is why I remember some of those first babies so vividly. I know it's why I remember Sarah.

Several months into that new job, in the middle of the night, I stirred with a slow awakening as the dark room melded into dream. A muffled sound emanated from down the hall. My tired body fought off the waking, but the sound was strange and different and couldn't be ignored. My wife and I rose together and padded down the hall, the front porch light streaming through a top window, bathing the hallway in pale light. The noise came from our youngest daughter's room and we crossed the threshold to find her standing wide-eyed at the railing of the crib, chest heaving, a croupy seal-bark cough gripping her. Her helpless eyes looked up at me as I scooped her into my arms and she gasped, "Help, Daddy." My wife and I rushed her into the bathroom, closed the door and turned the shower up as hot as it would go. But the steam was slow in coming and her breathing stayed heavy. Abandoning the bathroom, I slipped sweats and a fleece jacket on myself and a pink button-down jacket on her. I clutched her against my chest, and we descended the stairs and stepped out onto the back deck and into the coolness of the night. The cold seeped down the collar of my fleece and drew into our lungs. Sandwiched between me and my wife, her head found the crook of my neck, her thin brown hair falling straight, her serious pale face rounded with baby fat. After several minutes, the cool air calmed her inflamed airways and her cough subsided, her breathing once again quiet and calm. We stood with pale faces under a crescent moon, the woods dark across the lawn, and I was overcome with gratitude for my daughter's smooth breaths and her body between us. The simple remedy of cool night air and our presence soothed her; for the babies in the NICU it was more complicated.

As it sometimes does in quiet moments, my mind wandered to the list of patients I had seen earlier that day. That morning I had pulled into the hospital parking lot, the building several stories high and welcoming with its warm and unassuming red brick façade. Entering the NICU, I stopped at a sink to lather soap over my hands. Sparkling morning sun refracted into the bay windows, swathing the babies in light. Around them nurses bustled with syringes and small bottles of milk. I made my way from bedside to bedside, opening the side ports of incubators, gently peeling back the linens to listen to hummingbird hearts. In open cribs lay the larger babies, tightly swaddled, feeding tubes taped to soft cheeks.

Sarah lay in an incubator, a knitted quilt folded on top to dampen the light, her parents sitting beside her. Sarah's mother Lisa had eyes that shimmered, broad cheekbones, and midnight hair in waves. Her father Eli was short and thin-boned and quiet; his head was shaved clean, reflecting the overhead light.

Sarah shared the bay with three other babies. Across from her lay a jaundiced baby, surrounded by lights casting an effulgent blue. All day and night Sarah must have heard the monotonous click and rush of air as the ventilator for the baby next to her counted out its rhythm. If she could have seen through the thick condensation adhering to that incubator, she would have seen a runty, wrinkled form resembling a fetus.

It struck me how little I knew of Sarah's story. My rounding sheet told me her last name: Godwin; mother's first name: Lisa; gender: female; weight: 874 grams; day of life: 36; birth gestation: 26 weeks; diagnosis: prematurity, respiratory distress syndrome, grade one intraventricular hemorrhage. The sheet was silent about the undercurrent of subjective information: was the pregnancy wanted; had it been comfortable, or fraught with complications and stress? How were the parents coping in the aftermath of the unexpected preterm delivery, with the terror of seeing their baby fighting to breathe?

The rounding sheet couldn't describe the parents' ecstasy of hope when Sarah was stable enough to come off the ventilator, how they allowed the rays of hope to enter in, hope she might live.

Performing my daily examination of Sarah, I slid my fingers over the soft spot on her head, the sponginess giving way to the bony ridges at the periphery. I placed the metal rim of the stethoscope over her heart and lung fields, then on her abdomen, listening to the gurgle of her intestines. At the side of the incubator, a machine pushed air into a mask covering her nose, the air spiraling down her nasal passages, down the rings of her trachea, and into the grapelike bags of alveoli in her lungs. A feeding pump squeezed khaki fluid through a tube in her nose. She squirmed as I examined her, pushing uncannily strong arms against my fingers and shoveling the back of her head against the mattress; her skin was pink, and she was stable.

To my right, a nurse sat in a chair feeding a baby. As she tipped the bottle up, she gazed into the baby's gray-blue eyes, tiny creases sprouting from the corners of her own as she spoke to him. He had a short, nubby left arm with three rudimentary fingers projecting from the base and a missing right arm with a single finger emerging from the stump. Formula sat on his feeding cart in place of his mother's cocaine-laced milk.

A radio on the windowsill softly played U2's "Streets with No Name," transporting me back to a day in my childhood when I accompanied my mother, a district nurse, on her home visits. She navigated the streets of Wellington, New Zealand in an old Corolla, the radio playing that familiar song; windswept trees blurred past, punctuated by showers of red Pohutukawa blossoms and glimpses of whitecaps in the harbor. We entered old weatherboard homes on the sides of the hills, with dimly lit rooms and the sickeningly rich smell of roast beef and the sound of Tui birds warbling in the ferns outside. I looked on with apprehension as my mother rebandaged a leg ulcer, dosed medicine through an IV line, and assisted an elderly lady to the bathroom. My mother cheerily asked about their families, how they were getting on with the cooking and housework, and while they spoke, she unloaded the Meals on Wheels food into the refrigerator and counted out pills. There was something so kind, heroic, and selfless in her demeanor, and somewhere a seed was sown which would always hold sway over me.

That evening I signed out to the overnight physician, handed off the cell phone, and unclipped my name badge. As I drove home, the lake flashed past me, shimmering and shrouded in green. We ate dinner as a family in the dining alcove and afterwards my wife and I scrubbed dishes, then children; then there were prayers and kisses goodnight.

I didn't know it at the time, but during those night hours, Sarah grew sick. While I sat on the back deck with my daughter trying to relieve her croupy cough, undigested milk spilled from Sarah's lips and her belly ballooned into a taut globe.

The next morning, I stopped by the X-ray reading alcove before going to Sarah's bedside and peered at the dark lines of air running between the intestinal wall layers—a hallmark sign of intestinal inflammation and infection. A heaviness settled over me; I could feel it in my stomach and throat and pushing on my temples. Necrotizing enterocolitis, the words themselves ominous and sinister under my breath. I hated it like a foe; hated the way it crept up without warning; hated it for targeting the smallest, sickest babies and for the destruction it caused to the intestines—bacterial overgrowth, swelling, reduced blood flow, and sometimes death of both the intestine and the baby.

At her bedside it was as though a cloud had gathered, shadowing Sarah in a dampening gray. Her arms lay limp at her sides; her breathing was shallow and irregular, and her eyes were closed; pale blue threads of veins tracked across her protuberant abdomen. Sarah was like a baby from a World Relief commercial, emaciated arms and legs, bulging abdomen, oversized head on a thin torso.

Looking down at her body in the incubator, my stomach turned as I thought of the first patient with necrotizing enterocolitis I had cared for in residency training. I remembered standing over him, tubes and lines everywhere, tangling and entrapping. A small breathing tube was taped to the corner of his mouth and miniature clear bubbles oozed out over the tape. I remembered carefully laying a tiny stethoscope on his bare chest, his alarms protesting with flashes of light and loud beeps. Moving the stethoscope down to the convexity of his belly, I was struck by how silent it was, no gurgle of intestines peristalsing away, nothing but hollow silence. He died that night.

A decade later, I could still feel that same dread in my stomach. That morning I sat with Sarah's parents, the thrum of the CPAP machine in my left ear, the early morning bustle of the day about us. Eli sat unshaven and quiet. Lisa smoothed the wrinkles from her black skirt, her hands moving slowly and purposefully across the tops of her thighs. I wanted to reassure them, but as I looked at Sarah, I thought of other babies I had cared for with necrotizing enterocolitis.

I thought of emergency surgery performed at the bedside, the surgeon sliding the scalpel over the stretched abdomen, pulling out the strands of bowel and running it through her fingers like rosary beads until the pink ran into dark, dusky tissue, the excised bowel shriveled and wormlike in the small blue basin. I thought of the times when the bowel slipped out into the surgeon's waiting hands, the overhead light glinting off the black sheen, the entire length of the tissue a sloppy mess; tissue so friable it broke apart at the slightest traction. In those cases, there was nothing to be done. The bowel was scooped back into the abdominal cavity, the belly sutured shut. I thought of the times when everything happened so fast: blood pressure slipping, vessels leaking fluid, every organ shutting down. Of losing the heartbeat before the surgical table could be prepared, then sitting in the small conference room with the parents while grief collapsed over them.

The morning gave way to afternoon as the hours slid by. Sarah's breathing became irregular, the monitors howling at each pause. I breathed a half-formed prayer. We ushered her parents out into the waiting room, dragged a folding screen around her bedside, and fed a plastic tube down into her trachea. The ventilator counted out an even forty breaths each minute.

The sun dipped low on the horizon and I drove home, distracted, worrying about my daughter, wondering about dinner, worrying about Sarah and whether I needed to mow the lawn on my next day off. Such strange irreverent neuronal circuitry bouncing among life and death and the selfishly mundane all in the space of a minute. That night I slept with my wife's warm body next to me, my children twisting their sheets in their beds as they moved, our porch lights haloed by insects. Twelve miles away, the ventilator pushed air into Sarah's lungs, the IV pumps dripped fluids and medicine into her veins, and her nurse tended to her with stoic carefulness. In that incubator lay the promise of a giggling toddler, a young girl pretending to shave her daddy's face, a future of painted nails and bubble baths, the first day of kindergarten and years of expanding hopes and dreams.

In the morning, she remained in limbo. Her X-rays looked identical and her abdomen had the same tympanic, bloated appearance. The blood counts were stable, as were the vital signs. Her parents continued to sit, helpless, restless, and on edge. The day took no heed of Sarah's plight; the baby next to Sarah sucked warm milk into his belly and a father pushed a wheelchair bearing a new mother down the center aisle of the NICU.

There was nothing dramatic—the bowel did not burst nor the heart stop. For Sarah, there was just waiting—waiting for the disease to pass her by and leave her to grow and flourish or to take an even greater hold, delivering her to the operating room and quite possibly death.

Over those first several days her parents stayed beside the incubator while I followed X-rays and blood work. I softly pushed my fingers into her belly, trying to determine whether she was getting better or worse. Underneath my fingers, her intestines were under siege: fingerlike projections of villi, inflamed, swollen and sloughing off; bacteria translocating across the thin walls of intestine, leaching gas into separating layers of tissue—a sickening melting and obliterating.

Trying to determine the course she was on was like reading tea leaves. One day there was less of the frothy, bilious fluid that the suction gathered from her stomach; the next day, more. Her platelet level held steady, inched down, and then plateaued while her white blood cell count crept upwards. I stood at the bedside each morning, trying to recall the exact colors of her abdomen the day before. Was that hint of blue in her lower right quadrant new? For her parents, these signs took on a significance of mammoth proportions, a heartless journey in which tiny gains made one day were lost the next.

On the good days, when there was a small sign in the right direction, I felt unsure of how to respond to her parents. I didn't want to dampen their hopes or diminish their joy, I wanted to celebrate each miniscule change with them. Yet I felt a responsibility to stay realistic, knowing that at any minute her condition could deteriorate. I'd made that mistake before, answered the question, "Everything will be okay—right, doctor?" with a reassuring *yes*, only to have the ground shift. I had been guilty of being overly optimistic or foolhardy enough to think that I could predict the outcome. On those occasions, my heart tore as if I had broken a promise.

On the eighth day, brown particles floated in the trap leading from Sarah's nose; she rode the ventilator, never breathing for herself. She was still and flaccid, her abdomen distended and so blue it was almost black. We sat next to her. It was late afternoon. Eli refused to look at me, Lisa's eyes were damp and listless. It was time for transfer to another hospital for surgery. I ordered another X-ray before calling the surgeon. In the glow of the monitor, I squinted at the pixels, sure of what I would see, but instead her intestines were stable, no worse. Perhaps even slightly better. I held off calling the surgeon, drawing a new line in the sand: if she wasn't showing improvement the next day, I would call.

The next morning, she moved her arm as I examined her and tinges of pink showed in her coloring. It was like backing away from a ledge. I smiled at Lisa and silently prayed that Sarah would continue to improve. Incremental gains accrued until three days later, when I examined her, she responded, opening her eyes, squirming under my fingers and putting forth thin, weak mews. Her respirations, once completely reliant on the ventilator, took hold as she gained strength. Several days later, we slid the breathing tube out of her throat. Tenacious clear secretions strung from the bottom of the tube, which was tossed into the trash; the tube that had kept her alive for the past fourteen days lay amongst damp paper towels, empty flush syringes, gloves, and dirty diapers. For several long seconds her chest lay still, her eyes glazed, and her heart rate started to freefall while the saturation of oxygen in her bloodstream followed in tandem. I stood next to Sarah, steadying the mounting urge to take over for her, to bag air into her lungs and put the plastic back in her mouth. I wondered if it was a mistake to have removed the tube. Then, like a child riding a bike without training wheels for the first time, she caught on, sucking air into her chest, releasing the breath, then doing it again; an innate tidal rhythm.

Over the following days her abdomen gradually regressed, and less and less output tracked up the tube in her nose. Slowly, we reversed course, pulling the tube from her nose, stopping the antibiotics. Then, after almost two weeks, a minute amount of breast milk dripped down a tube into her stomach. Another week went by, the amount of her feedings steadily advancing, until she was no longer dependent on the yellow bag of intravenous fluids for her nutrition. Each day it became easier to talk with her parents; we smiled as we passed in the hallway, feeling a connection in having weathered the storm.

At the peak of her illness I had felt the breath of despair, dejection, and impotence on the back of my neck, cool and disorienting. It hounded me from patient to patient and from the hospital into my house. Later, looking at her pink skin, flat belly, and the slight crease of fat on her arms, I felt victorious. And yet I knew that we were fortunate. That no matter how hard we work, no matter how much expertise or knowledge or experience we pour into each baby, time will deliver a wide array of outcomes. Each day I will come home and set my worn black messenger bag in the mudroom, tell my family that my day was fine, and feel the privilege of being a part of those lives.

Several years later, I stood on freshly mowed grass, bathed in a warming sunlight while my son ran up and down the soccer field with his team. It was the kind of afternoon when everything seemed right in the world. Spring had transformed the dull brown of bare tree branches into a canopy of brilliant green. Even the tree trunks were greened by thick, creeping vines, twisting and cloaking. Over the green canopy expanded an endless vivid blue sky punctuated only by high-riding cirrus clouds. From the east, a faint breeze whispered in while birdsong tumbled out from the woods. Everything about the day spoke of rebirth and new beginnings.

As I stood lost in my own thoughts, I heard my name and turned to see a woman approaching with a toddler perched on her jutting hip. With so many babies moving through the NICU, I sometimes struggle to remember a patient's story. But when I saw Sarah's mother, it all came back immediately. Here was the vision I had needed to see years earlier: a chubby toddler in a white dress with lace frills, a pink bow in her hair, and a few delicate teeth. When her mother set her down on the grass, she lurched forwards into a run, plowing into my leg. I lifted her up. Her brown eyes searched me as I felt the solid weight of her in my arms. It was a lifetime ago that she had been sick, and this child bore no resemblance to that baby.

I smiled at her. "You're so big, Sarah."

She squirmed down and ran, until all I could see were the rise and fall of her feet in the grass, the bobbing of her black curls, and the pumping of her arms in the spring sunlight.

The Invisible Line

O ne morning during rounds, I received a frantic phone call from one of the nearby emergency rooms. The nurse yelled over the background noise and all I could make out was that they were performing a C-section in the trauma bay. I grabbed the heavy red jump bag, and the respiratory therapist and I set off at a run for my car in the parking lot.

It was just a couple of months after I saw Sarah at the soccer field, and I was still riding high. Although I knew I couldn't count her recovery as a testament to either our ability to save every baby or as a promise of future outcomes, it seemed only fair that I could enjoy some small portion of joy. Something to hold on to. Something to carry with me.

Outside the day was lazy and sultry, the sun not yet overhead. Past my window, green foliage blurred as I wove the car through sparse Sunday traffic, praying for green lights. The semicircle driveway in front of the emergency room was empty. I handed my keys to a security guard and jogged from the humid air into the thin chill of the waiting room. An elderly couple sat, leaning into each other, the woman's face pale. Across from them, a middle-aged woman peered into a cell phone.

I moved down an empty hallway, the sterile white walls impersonal. My shoes squeaked on the shiny linoleum, closing the distance. A nurse behind a desk looked up at me, a telephone wedged between her ear and shoulder.

Through the double doors, Trauma Bay 2 was awash in a sea of blue scrubs; a cacophony of urgent voices. Weaving through the throng, I came to the baby lying on a warming bed. Anna was blue and fat, her chest pumping up and down under a nurse's trembling hands. Another nurse poked the hollow metal of an IV into her pudgy arm. A respiratory therapist clamped a mask over the baby's face and squeezed a blue bag. The baby's heart did not beat. The IV would not start.

The emergency room physician came over to me. Behind him the mother's belly shook as her chest bounced up and down. Over her a young nurse, tendrils of brown hair escaping a flimsy loop behind her ear, pumped up and down. The doctor filled me in briefly.

"She collapsed at home. According to her husband she was doing the dishes, became short of breath, and then seized. By the time EMS arrived she was asystolic. They started compressions on-site but still no heartbeat."

"How far along was she?" I asked.

"Judging by her last OB visit, the baby should be pretty close to term."

"Did the baby ever have a heartbeat?"

"No. Nothing. No heartbeat, no respiratory effort. We tried a couple of times to get her intubated but kept ending up in the stomach."

The baby was now ten minutes old. Equipment was strewn over every surface: plastic wrappers, empty syringes, unopened sterile packs, used forceps, and scissors.

I was accustomed to resuscitating babies in the delivery and operating rooms of my home hospital where I knew the nursing staff and I knew my resources. Now I was in an emergency room across town, in a hospital without a NICU, surrounded by unfamiliar faces.

Pushing through drawers, the respiratory therapist found a new breathing tube, suction tubing, and flesh-colored tape. I slipped the metal of the laryngoscope between the baby's lips and in the pale light, bubbles of blood and secretions glinted and swam. The suction tubing gurgled and all I saw was pink floppy tissue. As I edged the laryngoscope back, the vocal cords flashed past me and were lost. I blinked, took a breath, and slid the metal in again until the vocal cords were there, swollen and motionless.

I listened to her chest while we bagged air through the tube into her lungs, hearing the fine crackles as her lungs expanded. Between the forced breaths there was silence as her heart refused to beat. Anna needed medicine. We squirted clear epinephrine down the breathing tube and squeezed air in as the fluid momentarily drowned her lungs. Next, I cleared a small metal table and opened a sterile line kit. I could feel eyes on me as time sifted away and the baby lay blue. I probed for a vein in the friable wetness of the umbilical stump, sweat meandering down my chest and matting my undershirt, the baby's body bouncing and the nurse puffing out the rhythm.

The clock's hand spun relentlessly. With each passing minute her brain was deprived of oxygen, suffocating the cells and wreaking havoc on the delicate machinery of her neurons. In the glare of the trauma lights and frenzied commotion of the room, it felt unreal to be entrusted with this moment; what transpired could last forever. There is an invisible line, different for every baby, for every family, beyond which the body can be saved but the neurologic injury is too much to bear.

As I looked down at Anna, my mind lurched uncontrollably, my stomach tightening with the anticipation of telling the father more devastating news—that in the wake of his wife's death, his daughter had brain injury or was also dead. I flashed back to a recent vacation to Disneyworld. In a crowd of people, I had seen a teenager with his parents, the electric wheelchair cleaving through the crowd, a high-pitched cry as his head twisted erratically and fingers clawed around the joystick. The sun was bright and brilliant and as I looked at the parents I had wondered—if they knew all that they know now, if they could go back all those years, what would they tell the doctor to do? To end the resuscitation sooner, to call the code and let the baby's soul flee from the brokenness? Then perhaps their marriage would be saved, perhaps there would be money for retirement, perhaps there wouldn't be the endless worry over who would look after him when they were gone. If I asked that question, would they blink in disbelief, incredulous and bitter at my lack of understanding? This was their child, no different in their eyes than mine are to me—loved, cherished, and protected, a wellspring of pride and tenderness. If Anna lived, would her future look like his?

The central umbilical line met resistance and a bubble of air rather than blood floated in the tubing. A voice from within, clear and cutting, wondered whether I could get the line this time; could I get the baby back? And if I was triumphant and her heart flickered and blood moved through the black courseways of her blood vessels and the ventilator forced oxygen into her lungs, to what end is that triumph? To send the father home with a baby who may need constant nursing care, to be fed with a tube; who seizes and never walks, never hears or speaks—no syllables, only grunts and moans? I make the decision over the course of minutes; the family lives with the decision over decades.

And then the line moved surely, cobalt blood in the tube. Clear epinephrine and normal saline and the heart jolted from hibernation. I took a step back and across the room I saw the obstetrician tying sutures along the gape of the mother's open abdomen. The floor seemed slanted, the noise garbled, the natural order shattered: the baby alive, the mother dead.

With the baby's heart beating steadily, I stepped out into the quiet of the hallway where the father sat on a bench. A window behind him cast him in light. It felt for that moment as if we were the only two people in the world. When he stood, his eyes were level with my forehead, his handshake enveloping. In a sports coat, collared shirt, tailored jeans, and dress shoes, he seemed out of place amongst the wreckage.

There was no good way to start so I opened my mouth and let the words fill the air, plowing before me. Sixteen minutes without a heartbeat, lack of oxygen to the brain, extremely high chance of brain damage. The space compressed, his head nodding slightly, while I felt small and weak, like a child holding out a broken gift.

From the periphery, an older gentleman emerged, distinguished gray-streaked hair, a rigid spine, intensely focused cedar eyes. In an instant, an unquestionable power dynamic emerged—standing with his shoulder angled slightly in front of the father, he spoke directly to me. He was the mother's father. Anxious to return to the baby, I left the two men standing in silence.

Minutes later I stood by the metal bumper of the ambulance in the emergency room bay as we prepared to transport the baby across town to the neonatal intensive care unit. An incubator was strapped on top of the stretcher, the wheels collapsing up as she slid into the back of the truck. Drops of maroon blood speckled the unisex blue-and-pink-striped blanket, her chest rising and falling with the ventilator and ugly pink cloth tape running out from the breathing tube across her cheeks. As I looked at her through the plexiglass of the incubator, I felt conflicted—we had saved her life, and I hoped that her brain would recover, but the guilt seeped in that it most likely wouldn't.

Over the first several days the waiting room was full of visitors for Anna. They filed into the NICU in pairs, replacing each other with knowing glances. The only deviation from the order was her father, who sat alone, staring silently at his daughter. In those early days, blood oozed from her mouth and her umbilical cord and any venipuncture site. The blood vessels in her lungs were tightly constricted; special gas from a chest-high canister pumped into them. Her kidneys were barely functioning. She had only scant bloody urinary output, her body was becoming bloated and swollen. At times her body twitched, her mouth chewing on the breathing tube until more seizure medication placated her irritable neurons and she became still. On my daily exams, I noted her puffy eyes, her pupils large and unresponsive to light. When I slid my finger down her throat, she did not gag. Her arms lay leaden and floppy. Her father sat, leaning forward. "Is she getting better?"

I paused and said that we didn't know yet, we hoped so, but it was too soon to say.

I thought back to a patient I had cared for during the first year of my pediatric residency. The first morning I approached the bedside and found her mother, holding a large baby in her lap. I hastily glanced at my sign-out notes: hypoxic ischemic encephalopathy, seizures, renal failure, pulmonary edema, oropharyngeal dysphasia, hypotonia, thrombocytopenia, anemia. I had little idea what half of the words on the sheet meant and yet with all the confidence I could muster I introduced myself, the words sounding suspect and more like a question than a statement.

"Hi, I'm Dr. Rattray, I'll be taking care of your daughter for the month."

Maddie's mother looked up at me with fierceness in her eyes. I remembered the nurse warning me, "Make sure you listen to the mother. She's seen a lot of residents over the past few months."

After wiping the bell of my stethoscope with an alcohol wipe, I pulled up a chair and slipped the end of the stethoscope down the baby's onesie so that I could listen to the pitter-patter of her heart. Having something in my ears gave me a few safe moments where I couldn't be asked a question and allowed me to observe my new patient. The short tether of the stethoscope drew me close and I could smell the curdled milk that leached from the receiving blanket and see Maddie's eyes slip back, revealing the white of her sclera. Under my fingers her skin stretched like a drum and when I put my finger in her hand there was no grasp; her arms were floppy and wobbly.

Her mother smoothed blond wisps of hair behind her ear. She intimidated me with her strong gaze, her black mascaraed eyelashes, high cheekbones, and diamond earrings. She sat with a bloated baby with roving eyes and slack muscles and raspy breathing and I was just one of a long line of young residents who knew nothing.

Pushing back the chair, I hid behind technical words, the plans for a *feeding advancement, electrolyte testing, weight adjustment of the seizure medication*. It was as if I had been dropped in a desert landscape with only a sliver of a map and no landmarks. Despite my detailed plan for the day, I couldn't see the big picture—I had no idea of what we would need to accomplish for Maddie to be able to send her home. As I spoke, I could feel the deep divide between her mother and me. She knew that I was there for only a month and that no one could help her baby to see or hear or heal her kidneys or reverse the brain damage. We couldn't change the future that would surely bring further heartbreak beyond words. As I looked at Maddie, I thought of my own baby at home with bright eyes, my baby who could sit up and babble. I thought of lying on a beach with him propped between my wife and me.

Guilt and helplessness hit me hard that morning and despite the passage of years, the same situations and questions still arise. I often find myself wondering what my role is. Am I a bystander, or do I somehow bear responsibility? I wonder if I could do more, show up in a different way? One thing I knew that morning when I first met Maddie and her mother was that I was on the other side. Not because I wanted to be but because I was only ever going to be a temporary figure in their lives. And perhaps worse yet, I was a part of the tribe that had failed to prevent this, failed to reverse it and never could. I didn't hold any kind of resentment about this—it's the nature of the mirage. I receive undue praise for good outcomes and criticism for things I can't control.

We didn't know it then, but her husband would soon leave her. I found out from the nurse three weeks later that he had an affair, moved out. He found a woman without a broken baby. I thought of how my wife and I rarely fought but when we did, it was about the dog who hounded our feet in the kitchen, or the way I snapped at her when she asked me a question when I came home from a thirty-hour call. I couldn't help but wonder what that kind of tragedy would do to us. Would we cling together or retreat into ourselves or lash out at each other? I know that I will find out the answer to this question in time—no couple can be entirely spared from heartache and I pray that I will be found faithful and steady.

Each day I drove back to the hospital, past the little white farmhouse with a faded American flag fluttering on the front porch, past the green fields with the cattle already huddled under a tremendous oak. Days melded together. I was busy and always behind. Anna's condition didn't improve, and an MRI showed all the signs of brain injury. She didn't breathe, and when her eyes opened, they roved erratically, lolling back in her head, revealing the white sail of sclera. When I spoke with her father he just nodded silently. I couldn't tell what he was thinking.

One afternoon during a lull in my work I pulled up a chair and sat with him, the two of us looking at Anna. Minutes dragged by and I fought the urge to jump up and get back to the endless paperwork.

"They all hate me, you know?" he said. The story slowly unfolded.

Ngoni was born and raised in Matabeleland North Province, Zimbabwe, near the southern bank of the Zambezi River. He worked as an accountant. One evening at his cousin's house, he met a young woman, Grace. She had traveled with her family from the United States to visit relatives. I listened as he described her—Grace with long black hair, gentle eyes, and skin that beckoned him. That evening they couldn't stop talking, and when she returned home letter after letter flew back and forth over the plunging jungle, the breakers, and the vast Atlantic, those words on the pages inroads to the heart.

Too soon, according to her family, he proposed. They were wed six months later. To her family it didn't seem right—the truncated courtship and a ticket to America for Ngoni. His Zimbabwean money wouldn't go far in the States.

They started a life together in a new city. Ngoni took an entry-level job in information technology while studying for the United States accounting exams. Grace worked as a nurse in a nephrology clinic. I could picture her as a buffer between her family and Ngoni—infusing light and joy, pressing the side of her hip against his, a reassuring hand on the back—a bold and carefree defiance. Now she was gone and all that remained was their broken baby girl.

Ngoni related that Grace's father and brother, mired in suspicion, blamed him for her death. They figured he didn't need her now that he was in the United States. It seemed to me the accusation was magnified and intensified through the lenses of mistrust, grief, and failed dreams. Now I knew why Ngoni always sat alone, why the grandfather grasped my elbow, leading me out into the hallway to talk alone, and why the air was thick with hostility when the family traded out places at Anna's bedside.

Me—with a wife and three healthy children, friends, neighbors, a church family—sitting next to a man eight thousand miles from home, his wife in a newly dug grave, his daughter on life support. I had nothing to offer—no treatment, no therapy. All I could offer was my presence and so we sat, our words few, looking at Anna together.

Two weeks later I walked out of the hospital as the sun sank below the tree line; I could hear cicadas shaking their maracas frenetically in the trees. Behind me the door clicked shut and euphoria bubbled up within me. I was leaving for vacation the following day. I felt intoxicated as the weight of responsibility slid from my back, the grief and heartache temporarily left behind.

One day later and six hundred miles north, I knelt on the tile floor in front of a large bathtub in my parents' house, light pouring in through the windows. A pink orchid in a glass vase sat on the side of the tub. My three children, their tanned bodies squirming and glistening with suds, played with the same bath toys I had played with as a child. Over the stereo an old album from childhood steeped me in familiarity. As I washed the sand from the children's toes, a kind of peace settled over me. In that moment, work felt distant; Anna was in the recesses of my mind.

Too quickly the vacation ended and a week later I headed back into the hospital for an overnight shift. Nothing had changed while I was gone. Anna with her tight curly black hair and full cheeks, her soft flawless skin, lay riding the ventilator, never breathing for herself. If it weren't for the breathing and feeding tubes, she could have been in a diaper commercial— her body intact, her brain invisibly ravaged. Four weeks after her delivery, it was evident she would never recover.

It had been arranged for her to come off life support that day, but the moment kept being pushed back. Now it would be a job for the night shift. Ngoni couldn't bear to be there. In the early evening we wheeled Anna down the hall to a private room, the respiratory therapist bagging air into her lungs until we were ready. Her lead nurse had driven in from home to be with her and now sat on a reclining leather chair. I lifted Anna into the nurse's arms where she lay with eyes closed, her body contoured to the nurse's chest. I looked around the room. Tears slid down a nurse's cheeks, running soft tracks through her foundation.

The respiratory therapist loosened the tape. The breathing tube slid out, a strand of mucus trailing the corner of Anna's mouth. On the other side of the wall a baby cried; a bus blustered past the window. The world outside the room continued oblivious and unchanged, yet inside, time became thicker. Anna's chest was motionless, her eyes closed without even a flutter beneath her eyelids. By the time I listened for a heartbeat it was gone.

When I called her father at home, he acknowledged the news, mono-syllabic and remote. In the quiet of the office with the night on the windows, I sat at the desk and rested my forehead against my hands, feeling hollowed-out and guilty. I hadn't saved Anna. I had prolonged her death. My efforts were for nothing. The place where life ends and death begins is difficult to discern. Sometimes we don't get a heart rate until twelve minutes and the baby does well, other times we get it at eight minutes and the outcome is catastrophic. Some families tell me that all they want is to take a baby home, no matter the level of disability, and other families tell me that they do not want to take home a baby with disabilities—for them, the outcome is too close to death. The line shifts and floats like mist. And I know that I will have to find forgiveness, forgiveness for inadequacy and failure and futility. I find my way haltingly forward.

Henry and Greyson

One morning, before going into the hospital for my call night, I worked in the yard, the warmth of spring on my neck and the air heavy with pollen. My daughter played in the sandbox, and the sight of her small form hunched over a bucket filled me with love and made me want to scoop her up and hold her close. Thankfulness and possibility welled up in me. And yet, as I worked, I felt an uneasiness as my mind wandered, subconsciously noting the hours until I was due at work. The anticipation of the overnight call cast a shadow. Little did I know that the apprehension I felt that day would be justified.

That afternoon, only an hour after changing into scrubs and getting sign-out from the day physician, I was called to labor and delivery. Afternoon light shone through the window, making puddles of white on the wooden floor. High on the wall, a muted television ran a detective show and in the center of the room Rebecca sweated through each contraction. Her husband, Colin, grasped her left hand, shifting from one foot to the other. On the other side stood Rebecca's mother, her slender fingers caught in her daughter's grip. Her mother leaned over her, counting. Under a spotlight the obstetrician sat on a stool, one hand on Rebecca's abdomen, feeling the contractions cramp down.

A labor and delivery nurse came over to the respiratory therapist and me to tell us the history. "She's here with twin boys at thirty-four weeks, we're inducing labor for severe preeclampsia. She's on magnesium, group B strep-negative, no prenatal complications."

While she spoke, we checked equipment. The valves hissed as we turned on the suction and oxygen, and the orange coils of the warmers glowed onto fresh towels awaiting each baby. Across the room a monitor picked up the fetal heart rates. With every contraction, the pauses between each beat elongated until the contraction passed and the heart rates surged upwards again. Rebecca let out small grunts and her mother smoothed her hair back off her damp forehead. People spoke in low tones that punctuated the quiet. After the equipment was ready, I stood to the side, waiting. My eyes were drawn to the out-of-place television, where a police car wove through Manhattan.

Ten minutes later, the first baby slipped out with a gush of fluid. He squirmed in the obstetrician's hands, waving his arms and kicking his legs, and after a ten-second pause, he wailed at his new surroundings. Under the warmer we dried his head, chest, and back as he cried, and the color seeped into him. Several minutes later his brother joined him, and they cried together under the lights of the warmers. We swaddled the babies and placed them in Rebecca's arms. She kissed them on the bridges of their noses and flinched as the obstetrician placed sutures through a perineal tear. I stood next to the bed, watching the babies' color and the soft rise and fall of their chests. It seemed that the minute hand barely moved and I kept glancing up at the clock, feeling guilty for my impatience. Even though they were breathing well I was anxious to get them to the NICU, as required by protocol based on their gestational age. I picked each baby off Rebecca's chest and placed them together in the transport incubator. As I lifted them, Rebecca sobbed, and her mother looked at me with tight lips.

In the NICU we lay each baby in a separate warmer along the same wall. After eight months of sharing the same tidal pulls, the same cadence of their mother's heartbeat, they were apart. In the new world they in-habited, everything was tracked: the peaks and valleys of their heart rate morphology, the rolling hills on the oxygen saturation monitor. A phle-botomist drew blood. The results showed normal blood glucose, normal red and white cell counts. We assessed them for oral feedings but when the nipple was placed in their mouths, their lips remained motionless for several minutes. Then they sucked and promptly sputtered, too immature to coordinate the necessary suck, swallow, breathe sequence, their oxygen saturations and heart rates dropping. While I wrote the delivery summary, the nurses floated feeding tubes down their noses.

During their first evening as parents, Rebecca and Colin sat in over-sized reclining chairs, a boy in each set of arms. In Colin's face I caught a glimpse of that feeling of newness and promise and responsibility that comes when holding a newborn, the feeling that the landscape has shifted and you would die for that soft sleeping face; that you are more vulnerable than you could ever have anticipated. The twins settled in, breathing reliably and tolerating the small volumes of milk we gave them through the feeding tubes. Day turned to night and the boys slept five feet away from each other. Every three hours, drops of breast milk ran down the feeding tubes, diapers were changed, temperatures recorded.

It wasn't until late the next morning that Greyson spat up, a small yellowish splotch on the sheet. At first, it seemed to be the usual premature baby spitting but as the day wore on, undigested milk seeped from his lips until everything we put down the tube came up. By lunch the monitor alarmed as his heart rate took quick little dips and his breathing paused. He was pale and didn't move, and when I pulled on his arms and legs they flopped back onto the bed. The light angled through the far window and seemed to pass right through the fine hairs on his cheeks and forehead; shadows formed between the valleys in his wrinkled brow. His eyes were closed, and for ten seconds his chest stopped moving under the stethoscope; I could hear each heartbeat separate out, the spaces lengthening and everything growing strangely quiet. I jostled him and they came together, the pace quickening. Within hours, he was unrecognizable as the baby we had admitted the day prior. He needed everything at once: central venous access, mechanical ventilation, antibiotics, fluids, and a diagnosis.

We cut the umbilical cord clamp from his drying umbilical stump and fed central lines through the vessels. While we worked, the pauses between his breaths elongated and his oxygen saturations banked down, rising and falling on an unseen current. Behind the mobile partition, his parents waited in the doorway, his mother in a wheelchair, his father standing behind it. The grandmother asked the nurse when Greyson could feed. I worked to suture in the central lines, the black thread winding around the supple lines as the monitor beeped incessantly. I thought about how this shouldn't be happening; the possible causes were seemingly endless. His saturations dropped low and we quickly intubated him before there was even time to explain the changes to his parents. As we worked, I sensed their presence on the other side of the screen, hyperaware of everything they must be seeing and hearing; the ventilator wheeling past them, our voices coming through the screen, the sound of the suction gurgling, the monitor shrill. After we stabilized Greyson, I approached his parents and grandmother in the hallway, conscious of how suddenly everything had changed for them. Rebecca stood with one hand over her still-protuberant belly, her face pale and gripped in an unconscious wince, her hair loose and dull and eyes glassed. She stood in the shadow of her own mother, her presence reduced, and she seemed to me like a young girl there at her mother's side. Colin mirrored his wife's meekness, standing in a crumpled T-shirt, the undersides of his eyes bruised and a rash of brown stubble covering his cheeks and neck. The grandmother looked at me with intense unflinching eyes, stalwart and protective. "Why can't he breastfeed?" she asked me. "He needs his mother's milk."

It felt as though there were miles between us. My words seemed to move around them, unintelligible and foreign. What I wanted to tell them was that I too was a father. Nothing I had experienced could compare to what they were going through, yet I wasn't a complete stranger to worry. I remembered the time my breath came in short little pulls when my son was born, and the brown meconium gushed out as my wife's water broke. The neonatologist suctioned the muck from his mouth and my son wailed. Several hours after the delivery of my second daughter the nurse checked my wife. Blood had soaked through the pads and her face was pale. The nurse excused herself to call the doctor. I wanted to tell them about these things, to close the distance, but my own experiences paled in comparison.

I led them into the room, standing to the side so they could see Greyson—their baby with a tube taped to his mouth, color-coded wires sprouting from his chest, a central line diving into his abdomen. He was still and gray. I thought of them at sea in a squall, blinking away the rain falling from a sky that only moments before had been clear and cloudless. I saw the meniscus of teardrops on the linoleum. My throat caught and I turned away, calculated the number of milliliters of normal saline to prop up his falling blood pressure.

Greyson on her right, Henry on her left. Why was one sick and not the other? I wondered about this question on two levels, first from a practical standpoint: what was different physically between the brothers? Did Greyson have a heart defect, sepsis, an inborn error of metabolism? Then there was the question we all ask of life: why does tragedy befall one person and not another? Every day we hear of people affected by earthquakes, hurricanes, and insurrection. One soldier dies and not another, a commuter dies in a car accident while the car next to him passes by unscathed. In our own circles, a seemingly healthy friend gets breast cancer. Just last week the medical transport helicopter I often flew on fell from the sky, leaving no survivors. I knew the crew. I look at my children and think, *that could have been me.*

I stepped over to the computer by the window to order blood pressure medication and soon more medication pumps flashed numerical green rates, making faint groans as they squeezed their contents into him: fluids, antibiotics, blood pressure stabilizers. I heard the lumbering of the ultrasound machine coming down the hall and looked on as the ultrasonographer scanned his heart. Jets of red and blue coursed through the grainy images; his heart's structure and function seemed good. Ten minutes later the cardiologist called to confirm that the study was normal. A new set of lab work emerged on the computer screen. His white blood cell count was low and new, immature white cells were being pushed from the bone marrow to fight an infection. As a child, I had a book about the human body in which the white blood cells were knights. In the picture, they spilled from a castle to battle invading germs. Now this battle was taking place before me, hidden from view beneath Greyson's skin. I stared at him and felt alone and powerless, his parents and nurse looking at me as I stood over his sick body.

We had done everything we could and entered the waiting period. Greyson was surrounded by tiny blinking lights like those in the cockpit of a plane: lights on the ventilator, on the monitors, on the medication pumps. Oxygen pushed into his lungs; blood pressure medication, antibiotics, and fluids into his veins. Greyson's mother looked up from Henry to where a couple across the room leaned down and kissed their daughter's nose, pulling her sleepy body out of the crib, offering her milk, and relishing her soft newness. Each family was vulnerable in their shared space and experience, their joy and grief laid bare.

Outside, the darkness came crawling down. The black curtained the windows and the hospital became lonely and isolated, an island unto itself. I went into the office to call home. My children each took turns telling me about homework, dinner, and baths. They were only twelve miles away, yet their voices seemed thin and distant. I wanted to hold them, to kiss their eyes and cheeks and lips, feeling the night stretching before me like an ocean.

I was in the next room checking on another baby when Greyson's heart stopped. I heard a call from the nurse, feet pounding the linoleum, and when I got to his bedside the heart rate on the monitor was flat. Placing the metallic rim of the stethoscope against his chest, I heard my own blood coursing in my ears. His chest was still and hollow. A nurse encircled his chest in her hands, squeezing sternum to vertebrae. I pushed first a bolus of normal saline, then epinephrine. Three nurses manned a red code cart, drawing up medicine. A respiratory therapist squeezed air into his lungs. The air seemed to have a weight to it; we knew he wasn't coming back.

Before I had time to call for his parents I looked up and they were there, standing behind a throng of nurses who parted wordlessly as the parents were drawn forward until they reached an invisible line just four feet from the warmer. They stood there expressionless and drained, their baby boy ashen and flaccid. Reluctantly, I heard myself telling them what they already knew. Rebecca crumpled to the floor with a thud. Nurses helped her into a chair where she sat, hair wild and tears on her cheeks. Colin stood awkwardly with one hand on her shoulder. Every few minutes I placed the stethoscope onto Greyson's still, mute chest and pushed more epinephrine into his bloodstream. I swabbed rusty iodine under his soft ribs, angling a stiff needle, probing for a potential pocket of fluid compressing his motionless heart. Everyone in the room looked on and the syringe was empty. Fifteen minutes had passed. Once again, I spoke to Greyson's parents.

"Please, please don't give up on my baby, please. Keep going, do everything. Please don't give up on him," implored Rebecca.

A rock obstructed my throat and my heart twisted—I would do anything to get him back, but I already had, and had failed. I wondered how anything could be this permanent, how I could be so profoundly powerless when it was my job to stop this from happening.

We continued our choreographed motions: more squeezing of his chest, more breaths into the small cavities of his lungs, more fluid and epinephrine into his midnight blue blood. Another few minutes passed and I placed the stethoscope on his chest for the last time, listening to the blood in my ears for a full minute, calling the code, noting the time on the wall clock. As quickly as it all began the room cleared, leaving only a few nurses to tidy up the scraps of plastic wrappers and empty syringes. My words to his parents came out thin and flat and hollow. Five feet away, Henry slept peacefully, oblivious to the noise and commotion and to how this event would shape his own existence. He would never know his twin brother and would surely feel that loss his whole life.

In the early hours of the morning I tried to sleep in the call room, tossing in a twilight state, my hip sinking deeply into the mold of the hospital mattress as light flowed in under the door and footsteps retreated down the hallway. The phone rang and I answered on the first ring. It was the microbiology bench reporting bacterial growth in Greyson's blood culture. "It's a gram-negative organism. We'll have sensitivity data to you in a day or so."

I placed the phone back on the desk and stared at the wall, thinking about Henry. Henry, the twin who had shared the same blood in the womb, passed through a birth canal colonized by the same bacteria, and now lay sleeping next to the empty warmer. I moved out into the light of the corridor, blinking sandy eyes, pulling down a hiked leg of my green scrubs. In the NICU I gazed down at Henry, his skin flawlessly pink, the faint creases under each closed eye. I heard the ebb of air, sucking gently into his nostrils before being released.

It was almost four in the morning and it seemed that daylight would never come. I ordered screening labs for Henry and went looking for coffee. An hour later the results came back, and it was as if I had opened his brother's chart. Just like Greyson, Henry's white cell count was low and his immature infection-fighting cell number was high. A mounting dread settled in as I realized that the events of last night could happen all over again. A nurse started an IV and I ordered antibiotics. I wanted to order up a double quantity, to take them off the timed pumps and push everything in all at once. I found his father at the bedside and tried to explain the lab results without worrying him unduly, my voice betraying me.

By daybreak, undigested milk seeped from the corner of Henry's impossibly smooth mouth. Then came the blinking of lights and constant beeping as his oxygen saturations slipped. The respiratory therapist taped nasal cannula tubing to his cheekbones, each threading towards the other to rise shallowly into each nostril. I stood incredulous at the bedside as the nightmare unfolded a second time. Henry's parents moved in a trance, his mother with bloodshot eyes, his father shuffling down the hall. Word spread among the staff, people speaking in hushed tones, on edge; knowing looks in the hallways; silent prayers and disbelief. Soon, the lab called again: the blood culture was positive for the same type of bacteria that had killed Greyson.

After signing out to the oncoming day physician I drove home against the flow of traffic, the day so bright and blue and full of promise that I wondered if the events of the night had been real. At home, I dropped my work bag next to pink flip-flops and a fluffy white dog with a ribbon for a leash. My daughter wrapped herself around my leg and I dragged her into the laundry room, where I washed the hospital from my hands. The rest of the family were seated over pancakes, morning light streamed into the dining alcove. After breakfast I collapsed into bed, hurtling into a bizarre and incongruent sleep, my neurons disentangling and reforming, processing and deconstructing. When I awoke that afternoon, my eyes were thick around the rims, parched and adherent. Inside my head the synapses were sludged and I woke with an edgy restlessness. After splashing my face with water, I logged into the remote NICU census—Henry was still alive.

Over the next few days, I was a wreck. I did my best to hide it from my wife and children but beneath the surface I was on edge, regretful, running the scenes over and over. I was plagued by the fear that the bacterial sensitivity data would come back showing the bacteria was resistant to the antibiotics that we had treated Greyson with. Surely, I should have picked different antibiotics or done something differently—but what? Obsessively, I slipped into the office to log onto the hospital record, checking the antibiotic sensitivity data with the feeling of compression in my chest. It seemed to take an age but finally the data came in: the antibiotics had provided good coverage for the type of bacteria that grew.

Nevertheless, my nerves were frayed and my patience with my children was short. I told my wife the story, but the heaviness remained. I thought about calling a friend who practices adult critical care medicine; perhaps talking with him would help. Instead, I did nothing and moved through the days. I had travelled this road many times and knew that the only thing to do was to keep on going. I knew that the acuteness of my emotions would dissipate with time, the rawness fading as new memories amassed.

It was impossible to know if Henry would make it. Every small sign seemed like an omen. Heart rate dips were surely the beginning of a downward spiral. We watched his breathing obsessively. Yet after three days, the darkness seemed to break. Henry cried for milk, and when we fed him, the milk stayed down. The monitor alarmed its last as his heartbeat grew strong and steady. We removed the nasal cannula, and except for the abrasions left by the tape marks, he looked perfect. Rebecca and Colin fed him on their laps, and I wondered what to say, caught between the relief of Henry's survival and the grief of Greyson's death. Eleven days later, the IV antibiotic course was complete. Henry's nurse slipped the plastic catheter from his vein and pulled the sticky electrodes from his chest, the monitor going dark. I watched his parents walk through the front doors of the NICU to take him home, could picture them walking out the front revolving door of the hospital to drive home with one empty car seat.

As they walked out of the NICU I thought of close calls and why one had died and not the other, of how they had shared the same womb and been exposed to the same bacteria. For some reason Greyson had become sick first, his illness an early warning for Henry. We drew screening labs before Henry showed symptoms; antibiotics flowed in Henry's bloodstream before we would have otherwise harbored suspicions that he was sick. Greyson saved his brother's life—an unknowing sacrifice that only a twin could make.

Rain on the Horizon

D uring those first few years after training, the sense of isolation I felt during the night shift never really left me. Much like my experience moonlighting during fellowship, the hospital where I worked had only a few physicians in the building overnight: an anesthesiologist, an obstetrician, and myself. Despite the presence of a neonatal nurse practitioner, numerous nurses, and parents in the unit, I was acutely aware that ultimately the responsibility rested on me. Even now, I have difficulty sleeping in the call room, tossing and turning and never really moving past a twilight sleep.

One Wednesday night in late fall, I lay on the sagging mattress in the call room. The thermostat ticked, and light leached through the edges of the door frame; I could hear the click of doors and the beep of the time clock across the hall. Turning from side to side, edgy and restless, sleep lapped up against me. Before me a windswept beach emerged, a cobalt sky ranged over a mirage of blowing white sand, and out over the breakers curved a meniscus of blue. I held my wife's hand, the whorls of our fingerprints pressed together, a hollow space in the convexity of our palms; threads of hair blew across her face, the horizon mirrored in her eyes. It all floated before me: the swirls of hot sand, sanderlings hunting the water line, and the tanned legs of my children darting in the surf. Sliding further into sleep, the beach disintegrated and my wife leaned over the bathroom sink, her eyes inches from the mirror. Her right hand flicked up against the blink of her eyelashes, each lash thick and black and separate against the white of her sclera, against the green-flecked iris. Her breath fogged the mirror and she pressed her lips together, concentrating. The shrill ring of the phone jolted me awake and my heart lurched as I fumbled for the glowing screen in the dark.

"Stat section for a thirty-four-weeker in OR 2, fetal bradycardia," an out-of-breath nurse said; in the background, I could hear rubber clogs striking linoleum, raised voices and hands hitting the metal plates of the double doors. I let out a sigh, slipped on my shoes, and stumbled into the bright corridor.

Outside the OR, people grabbed hats, masks, and shoe covers. I could hear the gurney coming down the hall on its route from maternity admissions—left, right, right, almost slamming into walls. I balanced on one foot, trying to slide on a cover.

Karen lay on the gurney watching the ceiling tiles as they passed like railroad tracks. Cool fluorescent light washed the color from her face and the paleness contrasted with her red bouffant hat. She had walnut-colored eyes, powdery, full cheeks with a faint pockmarked scar on the side closest to me. Her lips were thin and drawn. I could see the tawny nail polish on her fingernails as her hands folded over her abdomen protectively. With the shouts and closing doors and people rushing around, I pictured her swimming in a kaleidoscope of fear. Fear for the baby and fear for herself and fear that everything was moving too fast and that she was falling. I wanted to stop the gurney and tell her everything would be alright.

The double doors jerked open and the gurney rolled past the obstetrician, Dr. Singer, her ponytail tucked into a surgical cap, the mask ties drawn tight, disposable booties clinging to her calves as she washed at the sink. Inside the OR, the team pulled the gurney up next to the table and helped Karen scoot across. A nurse guided her into a sitting position on the side so that she was hunched over, her back curved forward, opening the spinal facets. She shivered or trembled into the nurse's arms while an anesthesiologist with silvered hair sprouting from under his surgical cap inserted the bevel of a 9-centimeter needle between her third and fourth lumbar vertebrae. Next, they laid her down and she breathed a mask full of gas while a nurse threaded a catheter into her urethra and Dr. Singer swirled iodine on her sensationless belly. As the anesthesiologist clipped the drapes to the IV poles, Dr. Singer held the scalpel like a pencil and drew it towards her. Just two minutes later her hands descended into the thin red puddle, grasped the baby, and he was out.

For a moment, he hung suspended in her hands, his head lolling forward, his limbs flaccid, and all I could hear was the steady beat of his mother's heart on the monitor. A nurse rushed him over to the warmer and we rubbed his back, then listened for a heartbeat that wasn't there. I held a mask over his mouth and nose and intermittently covered a hole on the T-piece, each occlusion pushing air down into his lungs. After thirty seconds I listened again. This time there was only the shiver of air as the breaths dragged through his bronchioles. Someone hit the emergency code button on the wall while I lifted his slack jaw with a laryngoscope and guided a breathing tube through his vocal cords. While the respiratory therapist looped tape around the tube, a nurse squeezed out compressions, counting under her breath. Over the next ten minutes we gave three doses of epinephrine until we heard the thrum of blood moving through valves, coursing through conduits—he was alive.

We loaded him in the transport incubator and wheeled him four feet over towards his mother and father. The OR was quiet now. The wheels of the incubator stopped short against an IV pole and Karen craned her neck around to see his face. I told them that he hadn't had a heartbeat when he was delivered, that we had put in a breathing tube and given medications to get his heartbeat back. Dr. Singer and a scrub tech continued their work methodically, sponging the blood, sewing up the horizontal gash. The anesthetist crouched over the urine bag, tallying the fluid level. I could see Karen's lips moving but the whisper was lost against the beep of her heart monitor, against the gurgle of fluid in the vacuum collection trap.

After we wheeled the baby into the NICU, I sat in the office, the yellow glow of the streetlights sifting through the slats of the blinds, the room silent. I thought about his physical exam, of how he lay unmoving, his arms and legs flaccid and leaden. He hadn't flinched when I opened his eyes and shone a light into the black, motionless pupils, nor had he flinched when I slid my finger down his throat—no suck, no gag. The ventilator initiated every breath. Running my finger down the therapeutic hypothermia protocol, I mentally checked off each box: metabolic acidosis, low ten-minute Apgar score, assisted ventilation, encephalopathy on exam. The only criteria he didn't meet was that his gestational age was less than thirty-six weeks—he missed inclusion by two weeks.

His neurologic prognosis looked grim. Within his brain a vicious cycle ensued. The process inside his brain unfolded like a story I read about from Iraq. It happened during the US occupation—crowds often gathered in the village square in the early evening, the air brittle with tension, heat enveloping the earth. Vendors set up food stalls with kebabs of lamb and beef, Qeema tomato and chickpea stew doused over rice. After the meal there would be chanting, the momentum rising as thousands of hearts beat together, lungs surging and feet stomping the dry dirt. Invariably, someone would throw a Molotov cocktail at a clay wall, someone would kick in a window, and the riot would begin. The sheer mass of bodies blocked the entrances to the square while the security forces on the outside looked for a way in.

A young army commander noticed the pattern: the crowd always ate before the ensuing violence. One day as a crowd built up, the commander ordered his security forces to stop the food vendors from going into the square. This time the crowd swelled and grew hungry as always, but when they looked for food, they realized the vendors were missing so people funneled from the square in search of a meal. Therapeutic hypothermia works the same way: cooling the brain is like starving the crowd.

It was 3:45 a.m., and I rubbed my eyes and paced the line of the office. I was faced with the decision of whether to follow the gestational age guidelines of the protocol or deviate from it. In medicine, every chance of benefit is tethered to potential harm. Exposing a preterm infant to hypothermia could trigger a pulmonary hypertensive crisis; could result in impaired blood clotting and bleeds in the brain, worsening the neurologic prognosis and resulting in a higher chance of death. Yet, therapeutic hypothermia could mean that one day he would feed from a bottle, crawl, walk, and perhaps even go to school. I thought back to my training. We had cooled two babies who were a few weeks below the age criteria. One developed severe pulmonary hypertension and we had to stop the cooling early, but the other baby had done well. As I paced the office I thought of the free radical damage, the excitatory cascade, the neuronal energy failure, and the chance we had to make a difference. I picked up the phone and called our medical director. He picked up on the third ring, his voice raspy and thick.

"Sorry to call—I've got something I need to run by you," I said.

There was a pause and I heard him shift upright.

"We just had a 34-weeker, stat C-section for fetal bradycardia. Got a heart rate at nine minutes. He's encephalopathic, initial pH of 6.8, base deficit of minus 18. On the vent and pressors. I'm thinking we should cool him."

I could hear him padding down the hall and he spoke in a high whisper so as not to wake his wife, "Okay, yeah—go ahead. Probably the best thing."

When the parents agreed, we would wheel a cooling machine the size of a mini fridge to the bedside, place a cooling blanket under him, slide a temperature probe into his esophagus and drop his body temperature from 37.5 to 33 degrees Celsius.

I found Karen and Jeff in the recovery room. She sat upright, her skin a flushed pink, brown hair falling over her shoulders. I knew instantly from the soft smile, the eager nod, the way she leaned forward in the bed, that a gaping chasm existed between her idea of her baby and the baby in Room 7, Bed Space 2. She didn't seem to realize how close we had been to calling the code, that on the ninth minute I'd thought I would tell them that their baby had died, that we couldn't get the heartbeat back, that we were so sorry, we had tried everything. Instead, now our feet trod in the no-man's-land of uncertainty. His heartbeat had returned and his lungs moved air, but the fate of his brain, starved of blood and oxygen for so long after delivery, hung in limbo. I looked at his mother, knowing that my words would most likely make no difference—her brain, soaking in endorphins, swimming with love for her son, existed on a different frequency.

And yet the gravity of the conversation hung over me. It could set the stage for the hours, days, and possibly weeks or years to come. The conversation does not get easier over time. Because I am going to hit them with a baseball bat. Punch them in the gut. Confirm every parent's greatest fear that something is not okay with their child.

Each parent approaches this conversation from a different starting point: some miss the gravity of the events and think their baby is doing well, while others withdraw, look anywhere but at me, shrinking back into the bed as if to prolong the seconds before I speak, to prolong the time when there is still a chance that they have misunderstood everything. In those moments I want so desperately to jump into the future, to see their baby five years down the road. How would I find him? In kindergarten, sounding through the words of *Green Eggs and Ham* and running across the playground, or at home in a wheelchair, deaf, blind, and nonverbal? I want to tell them what to expect and instead, the future is like fog on a Maine shore in the early morning—I can hear the deep, throaty call from the points of land but all I can see is swirling whiteness. Experience only thickens the fog by showing us that outcomes once considered a foregone conclusion can veer to the right or left: a baby who would be expected to die or suffer catastrophic disability toddles along during the developmental checkup, stacks the blocks, forms words, and receives a normal score. Another with a smoother hospital course may need physical therapy, speech pathology, may not eat enough by themselves and need a feeding tube. And always at four in the morning, with the baby only forty-five minutes old, there is a compelling need to say something, to make a promise to the parents who watched us wheel their baby down the hallway, away from them.

Karen looked up at me, smiling her soft smile and asked expectantly, "How's he doing?"

I drew in a slight breath, blinked, and tried to find a balance between optimism, hope, and reality. Stalling, I asked if they had given him a name yet.

"James," she said, the word carried into an ending inflection, borne on a smile.

"That's a great name. So, you know he had a tough start?"

She nodded.

"He didn't have a heartbeat when he came out, but we did the breathing for him and gave medicine to jump-start his heart. We got a heartbeat by about nine minutes of life." I held my hands together, rubbing my thumb over the boney prominence of the knuckle. "He's not breathing for himself just yet—the ventilator's doing the work for him. His blood pressure was low at the start, so we started blood pressure medication and it's holding steady now."

And then Karen dabbed at her eyes and Jeff squeezed her shoulder while I shattered their world again. I told them about the high likelihood of brain injury, comparing the brain to an injured muscle. Sometimes the muscle heals with ice and rest, and other times the damage is too great and it never fully recovers. There was no way to know yet.

When I looked at Karen, an inner voice wondered if I was overreacting, being overly pessimistic: could anything really be this bad? I shook off the doubts, thinking of James on the ventilator, unmoving. To say anything else would serve only to save myself from the pain and discomfort of delivering the news.

When does the need to do more, to intervene further, become something to hide behind? I have sat with parents, the monitors flashing red, their baby next to us in the incubator, his skin furrowed over bird bones, blood pooled in the ventricles of his brain, froth drowning the twigs of lungs, bacteria marauding the dark tunnels of his bloodstream and I know that the end is only hours away. As I sit there watching the tears slide down a mother's face, mascara drawing crooked lines, her lips trembling, I want to offer the world, every medicine I can order, every procedure I know to do—anything but admit that we have reached the point where doing anything further is prolonging their baby's suffering. Worse, much worse, is when the end of the long night is approaching; for an instant I might glance at the clock, as the selfish fatigue and emotional exhaustion bears down on me and hope that the baby stays alive into the next shift. After that will be guilt. Guilt at that passing thought, and later, guilt for leaving the baby's family while I change from scrubs to jeans, walk out of the hospital, and drive home to my own family.

In the smallest hours of the night, in the quiet of the recovery room with the blood pressure cuff on Karen's arm auto-cycling and Jeff shifting closer into her, I held out what little I had. We could cool his body for three days, then slowly warm him. I told them clinical trials had shown neurologic benefit, but their son didn't quite meet the age criteria. I explained that I thought it offered him a chance at the best neurologic outcome. Would they agree to it? As I asked them, it struck me how unfair the question was. I had spent a decade reading through the articles that spill from manila folders in my office and now in the middle of night I was asking these young parents to consent to something they had never heard of before; to consent for their baby when they had been parents for only forty-five minutes. As if it somehow removed some burden from us; as if, within the confines of time, knowledge, stress, grief, or euphoria we could adequately explain the recommendations. After fifteen minutes, my phone rang and I was notified that James's legs were bicycling, and his left arm was twitching. I excused myself from his parents and took the stairs two at a time back up to the NICU.

At the bedside I watched James's nurse lift him, his arms hanging down, his head lolling back, while another nurse slid the cooling blanket under him. The cooling machine hummed as it cycled icy water through the blanket; the baby's skin was stretched and shiny. He seized three times that night and I layered antiseizure medications until the movements stopped.

The morning light was slow to come but finally I could see the orange glow through the blinds of the office. When the day broke and washed away the darkness, it seemed that everything should start afresh—that nothing could be so permanent that the daylight couldn't make it right. I thought of how we should all get at least one retake, especially here in this country where we drink the power of positive thinking like thick, creamy milk and proclaim that everything happens for a reason, happens to teach us an important lesson. We even go so far as to say that God inflicts these circumstances on us either as correction or to teach us. I used to think this in a subtle, unrealizing kind of way; used to embrace that God. I watched a teenage girl with cancer spasm in the pangs of death rales; I listened to the fluttering heartbeat of an emaciated, bald five-year-old girl with a line of crimson blood curling down her nose and over the ridge of her lip. In the midst of these experiences something moved in me, something that built slowly over the years, layer by layer. Those were the days of a slow, burning resentment towards God. In church I recoiled at any talk of God's goodness. To me it was the lucky ones who spoke that way, and I felt alone and isolated by my experiences.

Later that morning, as James lay cooling in his incubator, I left the hospital and returned home, tired and spent. I sat in the kitchen, oblique sunlight warming my face and lacquering the table. On those post-call mornings, the emotions are contorted and magnified by my lack of sleep. For some reason I often think of friends that I trained with, those who stayed in the ivory tower of academia. Friends with laboratories, clinical trials, professorships, blue blazers hanging from the backs of office doors and offices that look out over the medical campus. Many of the night nurses couldn't pick those doctors out of a crowd—they never see them because it is the training fellows who stay in the hospital overnight. Those doctors lead studies that will change the way medicine is practiced and they will spend their careers fighting for dwindling grant funding, subject to cutthroat politics. Perhaps in some ways I feel less than them now. I work in a busy community hospital, spend all my working time in clinical care, stay overnight in the hospital. My suit is almost two decades old, the one I wore when I interviewed for medical school. Do other people feel the same way? Like it's never enough? No matter what we accomplish or do, there is always more. I look at my neighbor with the blue Audi SUV and a finance job and it seems to me that he has accomplished infinitely more than I. He waves as he drives past me in his sports coat, on his way to a corner office, while I drag the trash bin up the driveway. He's off to work and I will crawl into bed.

But then I think of an old Vietnamese grandmother I spoke to in the NICU that past week. Half the height of me, straight gray hair pulled into a long ponytail. The skin around her eyes was wrinkled and yet something, the smile in her eyes, gave her a youthful appearance.

"Do you have children?" she asked in halting English, tilting her head and looking up at me.

"Yes, three—two girls and a boy."

"They are very lucky to have such a kind doctor as a daddy."

And it reminds me too, of a crowded ballroom. I danced with two girls, one on my hip, her sweet breath on my cheek, the other twirling on my free hand. An older gentleman leaned over and told me I was a rich man, having those two girls. It was true and it checked me hard because of the amount of time I spent worrying about other things: retirement accounts, college savings, work schedules.

Isn't that enough? To be a husband and father? To care for babies?

A couple of years passed. A physical therapist came up to me in the hall one day. "You remember James Evans, right?"

I shook my head at first, then it clicked, "Yes I do."

"We just saw him for his eighteen-month developmental clinic visit. He's doing great, meeting all his milestones, looks perfect right now. Who would have thought? The parents are overjoyed."

I smiled and walked down the hall, memories of that night becoming crisp and vivid. I remembered the delivery room, the way James's straight brown hair matted to his forehead, that first night when he lay motionless in the bed, pacing the office trying to decide whether to cool him, and the late-night call to my medical director.

I looked out the hospital window. There was rain on the horizon, the tree line disappearing into an advancing darkness, the treetops undulating, crepe myrtles shuddering. Closer, the clouds had a complexity of color—ivory, dove gray, silvery edged, and pewter—until they melded into a solid slate gray that swallowed the trees. Time collapsed upon itself and I could see James that first night and imagine him now, toddling across a room. Turning from the window, I moved to the next bed space, slipped the latches, and reached the stethoscope into the incubator. A pink knitted hat cradling her head, her breath soft on my hand. The future always on the horizon.

Eleven Minutes

One year a local magazine featured a story about a family who was cared for at our hospital. Everything highlighted in the piece was true and my heart swelled with pride when I thought about the family and the role each caregiver had played in their story. But what it really made me think of was how few people know the entire story behind an event. Each person sees the same thing unfold from a different perspective—standing in different places, focused on their own tasks, seeing everything through their own lens. Sitting at the kitchen table and reading the magazine as I ate breakfast, the sun burning behind the height of the pines, I thought of my own recollection of what happened.

That afternoon, I hurried through the OR doors into bright lights and a cacophony of voices and frenzied movement. In the center lay the mother, Jennifer, the only still person in the room. Her abdomen gleamed white under the surgical spotlights; her face was veiled by the drape which rose vertically from her chest. The obstetrician, Dr. Turner, hastily poured iodine over Jennifer's abdomen, rivulets of brown tracking down her side and pooling on the white drape under her. Once the sterile drape was pulled over her, all was obscured but a square of skin.

"Breech, twenty-eight-week baby. Mom came in bleeding," an OR nurse called out to me.

A nurse led the father, Chris, behind the surgical trays and through the throng of nurses to the head of the bed where his wife lay awake, shivering.

Dr. Turner pinched her skin with forceps, checking the loyalty of the spinal block.

"Can you feel that?" she called to the mother.

The mother was silent. A second later the line of the scalpel ran horizontally across the gleam of skin. One stroke, two strokes, then marbled tissue gave way to the rice paper-thin amniotic sac. The scalpel slipped through the membrane and bloody fluid spilled out into the gullies formed by the drapes. Dr. Turner reached into the cavity, her hands probing as the stark lights sheened off the merlot fluid. Several minutes passed and still she couldn't pull the baby out—he was wedged down too low in the birth canal. For a sliver of a second her eyes met mine, then flashed back to the abdomen.

"I need someone to push from below," she called out.

A nurse crawled on hands and knees under the drape between the mother's legs and rummaged around.

"Are you pushing yet?" Dr. Turner called out.

"Yes—my hands are on him. He's not moving."

I could see the crook of the nurse's elbow jutting out from under the drape, blood tracking down her arm, dripping from the curve of her elbow onto her shoes. The obstetrician's hands reached deeper and I looked at the clock, my chest tight.

She shook her head. "I'm going to have to deliver this baby vaginally."

Once again there was a flurry of movement as she moved down to the base of the table and a nurse took each of Jennifer's legs, flexing them up and out.

While they worked, I thought about the abrupted placenta which had surely detached from the uterine wall—the baby's lifeline severed. Each minute the baby went without blood flow or oxygen, the chance of brain injury or death increased exponentially. No one could know exactly when the placenta had detached and all blood flow to the baby ceased. It could have happened immediately prior to the cesarean section when the vaginal bleeding started. Perhaps it had only partially detached at that point, holding on for precious minutes until a full detachment occurred during the operation. I glanced over the resuscitation equipment again. The respiratory therapist next to me shifted from one foot to another, her finger on the timer button of the warmer.

"I've got the neopuff and breathing tube ready for you," she said.

"Thanks," I said, feeling like a runner about to be handed a baton. In those waiting moments anticipation does strange things to me. I am drawn to the details around me. The print on the CPAP masking reads: Fisher & Paykel Healthcare, East Tamaki, Auckland; the surgical light is a bed of alternating blue and white spherical lights. I don't know why it happens, but I think these details keep me calm as I stand there, waiting to play my part while the emergency erupts around me.

More time, and then a collective murmur ran through the room as a pair of legs emerged, blue and bruised. With more traction came the torso and arms, inky and toneless. It was then that I realized his head was stuck. Dr. Turner pulled the baby's body from side to side, his neck elongating sickeningly within the noose of the cervix, thick and muscular and unyielding. From the head of the bed, I could hear soft moans at each pull.

Again, Dr. Turner looked over at me and for a second our eyes locked, hers with a wild desperation, mine with total helplessness—there was nothing I could do but stand there. She pulled on the body, working different angles, trying to get her fingers inside the cervix to loosen it, but there was no give in the muscle.

Suddenly a story came to me, one an older doctor told me a long time ago about a baby whose head became stuck and finally the only thing they could do to disengage him from the mother was to decapitate him. I thought of all the things I had seen over the years, all the close calls, but this held the promise of being the worst. If this happened, I knew I would never be the same.

When it seemed that all hope was lost, Dr. Turner grasped a thick pair of scissors and worked the blades on either side of the cervix, the muscle giving way in ragged strands as she squeezed the handles together. The next second, the baby shot out onto the bed, limp, blue, and floppy. Dr. Turner scooped him up and ferried him across to the warmer, almost throwing him at us in her urgency.

Only twenty minutes earlier I had sat at the desk in the office, twenty-eight progress notes staring at me from the computer screen. My eyes had felt like sand; the minute hand on the clock moved in small jerks. Standing to stretch, I gazed out the window and across the hospital parking lot. Roiling clouds hung heavy over threadbare trees, the afternoon light diffuse. I cracked open the window and sharp air surged into the room carrying with it the faint metallic taste of winter.

The task at hand stretched before me. The details of each baby had to make their way into the medical record: the daily physical examination, medications, respiratory support, type and quantity of feedings, new laboratory results, number of antibiotic days. By the end it seemed that each infant had been reduced to a string of data. Reading back over the note I had just finished, I could hardly tell which baby it was describing. As my fingers tapped the keyboard, I found myself wanting to pause time, to imagine it was summer and I was lying on my back under the elm trees that line the parking lot, a brilliant blue sky over me. I could sense that stillness. No cars or people passing by, no phones, my new world uninterrupted and unrushed. I thought of how I would go to the hiking trail that skirts the lake, time standing still, the earthy breeze shrugging over the water. I knew exactly the fallen log I would sit on in the alcove of sand, pondering whether to hike further along the shoreline or slip into the water and make for the island.

I ate a late lunch at the computer, trying not to drop crumbs between the keys, while I kept up the typing pace. Mid-note, my pager blared—they were calling me to an emergency cesarean section. After spitting a mouthful of food into the trash I started off down the hall, my badge slapping my chest, my toes curling slightly at the end to keep my clogs on. As I jogged I couldn't help hoping, with all the strength of selfishness, that the baby would be healthy and that I would be able to get back to my computer work and make it home in time to have dinner with my wife and children.

Outside the double doors of the operating room an empty gurney lay against the wall, a crimson halo staining the sheets. As I pulled on a hat and tied mask strings behind my head, I saw a man sitting outside, waiting to be called in after the mother had been prepped. He wore a hospital-issue white jumpsuit, a surgical hat pulled down too far, and a mask loose at the bridge of his nose. Through the thin white of his jumpsuit I could see the line of his shorts and, sprouting from the shoe covers, the rims of his Converse Chucks. He sat alone as if forgotten, as people streamed past him, voices raised and harried. With anxious eyes, he watched a nurse slam back out through the door and run down the hall, the heavy rubber of her clogs dull against the linoleum. I could feel the crush of time but reached out to shake his hand, introducing myself.

"I'm Dr. Rattray—I'm going to take care of your baby after he's born."

"Chris Walsh," he said, his hand enclosing mine. "Do you know when I can go in?"

"No, but they'll call you in as soon as she's all set." I wanted to say what I could not: that everything would be okay. Instead, I told him what I could: that we would take good care of his baby. Now, as I stood over the baby on the warmer the room was quiet, the unnatural silence of the baby hanging heavy. He did not wail; there was no soft lub-dub of his heart valves. Perhaps there were voices around me, but I did not hear them. All I heard was the silence in the baby's chest and all I saw was the color of his skin, the violent hues of a breaking storm. I fed a breathing tube through his motionless vocal cords, bagging oxygen into his lungs, listening to the sound of his sticky premature lungs inflating with the breath and the ongoing silence between breaths—not even the flicker of a heartbeat. One nurse compressed his sternum, counting the rhythm under her breath while at her elbow a nurse practitioner guided a catheter into his umbilical vein. I called for epinephrine into a crowd of nurses manning a red cart and a hand reached over my shoulder with the syringe. I screwed the syringe into a side port of the breathing tube and squeezed the stopper. The fluid trickled down the tube, then flashed back up again as it transiently flooded his lungs. The nurse paused compressions, listened, and shook her head.

When the umbilical catheter was in place, we pushed epinephrine and normal saline. I stole a glance at the parents, but the angle of the drape obscured the mother's face and only the father looked back at me. He sat six feet away, his expression hidden behind the surgical mask, his eyes steadfast and unblinking. The next dose of epinephrine wasn't due for another three minutes. Three minutes—time enough to anticipate looking into the father's and then the mother's eyes to tell them that their son was dead. Time enough to think of all those months of hope, shattered. I tore my eyes from the father, back to the baby on the warmer. With each compression the supple bones in his rib cage flexed in and drops of blood oozed from around the umbilical catheter; I could hear the bag crunch down as it squeezed air into his lungs. Three minutes later I listened again to the stillness in his chest. We gave more epinephrine, fluid, chest compressions, and breaths of oxygen. The clock on the warmer counted the minutes. Again, I glanced over to the father. From behind me, wisps of smoke rose as Dr. Turner cauterized the mother's bleeding vessels, the burned grease smell leaching through my mask.

Ten minutes had passed, and we were nearing the end of the code. The chance of getting him back was minuscule and even if we did, catastrophic organ and brain damage were almost certain. One more dose of epinephrine and I listened again. Then, where there had been silence, came a sharp, clear pulsing—so loud and sure as to always have been there. The clock on the warmer showed eleven minutes. The pulse oximeter picked up a signal. I inhaled through my mask and waved the father over. He navigated past the blue sterile drapes to stand tall over the warmer bed, mask reaching to hat, leaving only the bridge of the nose, eyes, and a thin rim of forehead. Creases sprouted from the corners of his eyes. I couldn't tell what his expression was, a smile or a wince of fear. He stood, massive, over his tiny son, seeing him for the first time after the months of feeling him turn and kick his hand. Now he could place a thick finger in the palm of his hand and feel the damp softness—he was a father.

"What's his name?" I asked.

"Joseph. After my wife's grandfather."

"Congratulations," I said, a strange remark given the circumstances, but I meant it—he had a son and his son was alive. "He gave us a tough time at the start. When he came out, he didn't have a heartbeat and wasn't breathing. We had to put in a breathing tube and do chest compressions, but now his heart is beating just fine. As you can see, he's little and sick. He went for eleven minutes without a heartbeat so unfortunately, he's at high risk for brain injury. We're going to show him to mom and then get him up to the NICU."

We lifted Joseph into the transport incubator, reconnecting the breathing tube to the ventilator and covering him with a warm towel. The incubator maneuvered into his mother's line of sight while her eyes welled and the fingers of her strapped-down arm reached for him. A minute later we wheeled away from her, the caustic sound of her retching trailing behind us.

Outside the OR, Chris ripped off his hat and mask, slumping into a crouch against the wall. His face was pale, eyes distant, one hand smoothing back over his hair. We waited a minute before helping him up and moving down the corridor, the four wheels swiveling under the plastic box. The fluorescent lights cast an uneven glow from overhead and the worn linoleum stretched out before us. Chris trailed a few feet behind and I turned to him in sympathy. "That's a tough way to start as a dad."

"The smell in the OR triggered my PTSD. It's like being back there—in Afghanistan—the smell of burning flesh."

It felt as if the air had been sucked out of me. To have seen him that way, hunched against the wall, his eyes staring straight ahead as he breathed into his hands, trying to shake the sensation, filled me with shame. That afternoon, all I wanted was to get through my progress notes and go home for dinner with my family. Now I could see how privileged and sheltered I was, how petty and selfish my desires were and how different my life was from this father's. It struck me how little we know of each other.

We were silent in the elevator; I had lost any ability to make small talk. And when I brought Joseph into the NICU all I could think of was: eleven minutes. What was the chance of survival, and what would be his quality of life if he did survive after that length of oxygen deprivation? I brought him into the NICU bay, not with the grin of a victor but with the sodden heart of one who wins a war in which much is lost. I thought of the spiderweb tangle of blood vessels in his premature brain and the way that, surely, they had burst during the fluctuations in blood pressure which occurred during placement of the breathing tube, chest compressions, or the boluses of epinephrine and fluids that we had given in the delivery room. A silent break in the tunnel wall and the blood would spill out into the surrounding brain tissue, red, caustic, inflammatory—toxic to the callow neurons.

At the bedside, Chris was even larger than I remembered from the OR, solid and stubbled, bending over to peer through the plexiglass at his son. Joseph lay nested in rolled blankets, bubbles oozing from around the breathing tube, his spindly arms and legs motionless, cobalt filaments of veins tracked haphazardly under the surface of parchment-paper skin. Above him, the lines on the monitor tracked along in various waveforms: his heart rate, saturations, blood pressure were all stable. An hour later, the overnight physician came in to take over for me. Before I left I passed back through the NICU, shook Chris's hand, allowed myself to smile, and headed for the door.

The next morning, I saw his mother at the bedside, and she looked entirely different. The day prior her face had been pale, her fingers trembling, her body laid out on the OR bed. Now, she stood with only a slight bend, the wheelchair behind her, her face full and flushed, one hand reaching in through the porthole of the incubator. I asked her how she was feeling, thinking of the way the scissors had sheared through her cervix.

"I feel pretty good," she said, her eyes anchored to Joseph. "How's he doing?"

"He's doing okay—all his vital signs are stable and we're not having to use too much pressure with the ventilator to support him. The amount of oxygen he is needing is really low, which is great. He's not out of the woods by any means, but he is doing really well—much better than we expected given his rough start."

She just nodded, smiling at him, her hand on the back of his. When I looked at him, I worried about all the invisible things she couldn't see or anticipate: intraventricular hemorrhages, white matter injury, respiratory distress syndrome, bronchopulmonary dysplasia, overwhelming sepsis, retinopathy of prematurity, necrotizing enterocolitis. She seemed not to see any of it. When she looked at him, she saw her son.

The first day came and went, and with each day the footing seemed a little surer. Joseph remained on a ventilator for several days before weaning to CPAP, then to a high-flow nasal cannula, and then finally to room air. The ultrasound scan of his brain showed the normal contrasts of white and black without the smudge of a bleed. He tolerated feeds given by tube and then started learning to feed by mouth eight weeks after his birth. During those weeks, the roses came to bloom on either side of the steps leading to the front doors of the hospital, green buds bursting into a lush blanket over the city. At home I mowed the grass, trimmed bushes, and relished the stray cool breeze on my face. As spring transformed the landscape, time and substrate transformed Joseph. Inside his chest the branches, twigs, and buds of his lungs matured while the smooth cortex of his brain wrinkled and furrowed into valleys and canyons. As the surface area of his brain increased, the magic of memory, learning, and cognition took hold. The routine of feeding, changing diapers, and administering medication went on, while hidden under soft skin and emerging fat rolls, the miracle that had started all those months ago with just a few lone cells continued.

Every day we tracked his weight, adjusted his feeding volume, titrated the medications he was on, and watched the fat turn him into a pudgy, kicking baby. Joseph's parents were frequently at his bedside, his father most often before or after work, his mother during the day. Over time, people forgot the way he had entered the world. When they looked at him they saw a healthy baby who was learning to feed, but when I walked past his crib, that first day in the operating room flashed before me and I knew how close we came.

His due date neared, and he was ready to go home. The night before discharge, Chris and Jennifer stayed with him in a private room attached to the NICU. Despite how long he had been in the hospital, it was the first time they were alone with their son, sleeping beside him, waking to feed him, and coaxing him to take his medicine from the nipple. The next morning, I entered the room to check on him. Light crested through the blinds, a breakfast tray sat on the table, and the room smelled of syrup and bacon. Jennifer sat up in bed, her hair uncombed, feeding Joseph. The door to the bathroom was ajar and I could hear the sounds of Chris brushing his teeth.

I felt oddly out of place in the homely familiarity they had built overnight—it was as though I had stepped into their house unannounced.

"How was the night? Did you get any sleep?" I asked.

"It was really good," she said. "He woke up every three hours or so, then went right back to sleep." In her arms he looked healthy and vigorous, with tight, curly hair and chocolate eyes.

"Wow, what a good baby. I guess you're planning on keeping him," I joked.

An hour later I was rounding in the hallway when Chris and Jennifer walked out of their room and down the main hall together, Chris holding the car seat between them. Jennifer was radiant in her joy, Chris strong and proud. They had weathered the storm and emerged intact. After all those months, Joseph would feel the sun on his face, take a breath of fresh air, and experience a myriad of new sights and sounds. He would wake up in his own crib, to his own parents. I wondered what kind of boy and man he would become, what his life would hold, and if it would somehow be shaped by how close to death he had come.

Pictures

I t was late in the day and I still had a handful of notes to sign. I was hoping to get the consult done quickly so I could sign out to the oncoming doctor, pass the cell phone, and finish up the rest of my work in time to take my nine-year-old son to soccer practice that evening.

I found Lindsey Marshburn alone, propped up in bed, the bedsheet pulled to her waist. Shaking her hand, I could feel the thin hardness of the IV tubing in her vein and I noticed the lean muscles of her arms, like those of a yoga instructor. Her pigtails and small, silver-studded nose ring conveyed an artistic openness to the world. It was Tuesday, the day after she had been admitted to the hospital and I was there to talk about what to expect if she delivered early. A lab cart rumbled down the hall and the hospital operator requested that the owner of a black Dodge pickup move it from the ambulance bay. Lindsey's phone rang and as she answered I glanced around the room. She had spent only one night in the hospital yet it looked as though she had been there for weeks. The afternoon light came in, backlighting photographs taped to the windows: pictures of a curly, tow-headed toddler running across a lawn; pictures of the same boy working his way across a driveway on a tricycle. In another picture, Lindsey held the toddler up to her face, his eyes blue and eyelashes long, his nose lightly freckled like his mother's. Around the room were traces of home. On the ledge under the window were kiwi fruit, a box of granola bars, a DVD of *The Notebook*, a set of folded pajamas, a hair dryer, and a laptop. On the nightstand she had arranged a pink journal, hair ties, and the same kind of lip balm that sits on my wife's bedside table.

"Sorry," she apologized. "My husband needed to know where my son's pull-ups are."

She told me, "I had a gush of fluid yesterday morning. I thought I'd peed, but I kept leaking so I went into the OB's office." She gave an uncertain smile. "They said my water had broken and sent me here—I know I'm early."

I smiled, hoping to convey reassurance and caring before launching into my routine talk: the baby would need help breathing, most likely needing a breathing tube, surfactant medicine to help the lungs. I paused. "Do you know if you're having a girl or a boy?"

"A girl," she said, glancing reflexively at the bulge of her abdomen.

We talked about the NICU, the incubator, fluids and tube feedings, the benefits of breast milk, the expected length of stay, and the complications of prematurity: chronic lung disease, brain bleeds, necrotizing enterocolitis. How many times have I said these words? How many times have they provided adequate preparation? What possibly could?

After I finished, she glanced at the pictures on the window. "They're keeping me here until I deliver. My son can't visit because of the flu restrictions—I've never even spent a day away from him before."

I thought about how when my son was a toddler, he only wanted my wife. I thought of the time she went grocery shopping and left him home with me and he stood at the window, watching the car backing out of the driveway, wailing.

When I think back on our conversation now, I have irrational, guilty thoughts. That I should have done more to close the distance, gone across to the nurse's station and dragged in a chair, should have sat down and shown her my own photographs. I could have shown her the most recent family picture we took, the one with our small sailboat tied to a tree on an island on the lake, my oldest daughter in a neon life jacket, her blonde hair falling down over her shoulders and the white line of her smile broken by the black of two missing teeth. At her side, my youngest daughter, a big proud grin on her face. My son with his arm resting on his knee, hair in a wave and a three-quarter smile. Me wearing a faded baseball cap and Wayfarers, and my wife with her hair caught in the breeze and a smile that radiates goodness. Instead, I stood in pine-green scrubs, a name badge dangling from my front pocket, a black phone clipped to my hip, and the patient list in my back pocket. On the back of that list was my thin, compressed handwriting, reducing her story to scrawled data: "Rm 301, Marshburn, Lindsey, 28-year-old G3 P1, PPROM, 23 1 wks, latency antibiotics, betamethasone x 1."

Maybe she thought she would make it to term. Maybe she thought this wasn't really happening, not in a definite way. Perhaps, as the weeks passed, she would drift off to sleep in the late afternoons only to wake up drowsy and listless. She should be combing through her recipe book. She should be rummaging through the vegetable drawer, taking inventory. Instead, there were sheets that smelled of bleach and slipped from the plastic mattress cover. I could only imagine the difficulty of her hospital confinement, how she must have longed for home.

Maybe she thought of her husband and son sitting at the dinner table, the early evening sun softening, her toddler dipping chicken nuggets in ketchup, leaving blobs down the front of his T-shirt. Now her husband soaping down the boy's curly hair, breathing in soft skin and baby soap. Perhaps, before he went to bed, she held her phone to her face, talked to the images of him, wanting to reach through the glass, to wrap him up in her arms and bury her face in his curls.

Maybe she showered quickly each morning, praying her cervix would hold. Maybe, as the TV flickered in the late evening, the heating vents periodically rumbling and muffled conversations floated past her door, she imagined before her hours that seemed like fog, obscuring beginning from end. She could swing her legs over the edge of the bed, plant her feet on the linoleum, walk down the hall, press the button for the elevator, and four minutes later taste the smoky haze of autumn. She could hail a cab and ten minutes later stand before her own house, the light coming from the windows, fallen leaves on the front path and sidewalk chalk left out on the driveway. Two more minutes and she could be in her husband's arms, then curled up with her son on the little toddler bed. She could run her fingers through his cowlick, down the curve of his back.

Five weeks later, I'm standing at her daughter's bedside, the moon hanging just over the roofline. I think of how the placenta had detached from the uterine wall that morning. Blood everywhere. Emergency C-section. Ava's hair is brown and downy and her eyes flutter beneath her eyelids. Her nose melds into rawboned cheeks, tape tracks across the corners of her mouth anchoring the breathing tube. Her chest vibrates in time with the hum of the ventilator. Her arms and legs are smooth and unblemished. Her knuckles are dimpled, the fingernails translucent. The diaper swallows her hips and is folded down along the top to make room for the IV lines in her umbilicus. Pumps flank the foot of the incubator and green pixels float across the miniature screens—medications and drip rates. Affixed to the head of the incubator is a pink sticker with her name Sharpied onto it.

I stand with the incubator at chest height. Ava is helpless. Machines squeeze medicine, glucose, fluid into her bloodstream; machines squeeze air into her lungs; machines display her heart rate, respirations, and oxygen saturations. Nurses connect IV lines and program pumps, nurse practitioners and doctors calculate drip rates and order medicines, pharmacists mix medicines, and technicians feed the liquid into syringes. Every minute, the monitor to her left emits a shrill alarm and I jab at the silence button until another minute passes and it starts back up. We adjust the blood pressure drips, the ventilator pressure, even try squeezing the breaths in by hand but the oxygen saturation monitor still flashes and beeps low.

Five hundred yards away is the Thai restaurant I took my son to several nights ago. We sat by a small wishing fountain with pink floating petals and looked at the bronzed deer headdresses on display, the delicate tones of the lute pulling us out of the strip mall, drawing us nine thousand miles away. I ate hot curry and drank a Thai lager. My son twisted darkened rice noodles on his fork, picking through green peppers and chopped onions. I wonder at the proximity of these spaces, at how little distance separates one world from the next. One night I'm a father, eating dinner with my son; the next, behind the closed doors of the NICU, I'm trying to keep Ava alive. Her nurse tends to the computer, entering vital signs, and the respiratory therapist moves onto the next room, rubber soles squeaking down the hallway. I think of the lung vessels in Ava's chest, like pruned tree roots, simple and thin. To my left a four-foot-tall tank bleeds gas into her lungs. The molecules cross the alveoli into her blood vessels which, in their oblivion or disinterest or apathy, remain constricted. Failure. Her heart squeezes against the tide, flagging, panting. Failure. Bluish blood lumbers through her overtight pulmonary vessels, those mutinous and unyielding vessels. I am angry at their obstinance. A decade of training. Failure. I run the lists in my head, arrive each time at a bricked-up door.

I wish I were waking up in a rondavel in the highlands of Africa with wisps of a smoldering fire melding into the morning mist, a cold stiffness in my bones, and a soft wind crescendoing through the grass. Let me see a baby with pneumonia, give a sticky pink elixir, approximate the edges of a laceration, give 75 milligrams of albendazole for a parasitic infection. Let me see one hundred patients. Let me be lost in the work, free of the electronic health record, free from the business of medicine and the commodity that

I have become. Let the plane leave me another night. I want to work with my hands instead of just watching the monitor helplessly. I want to throw myself into something I can fix. But I know that tonight I will tell Ava's parents that we are doing all that can be done and that all we can do is wait.

Hope is oxygen, sunlight, water. Hope is the way strands of light thread through the black shoulders of the clouds; the soft, familiar press of a daughter's lips after a day of work. What do I have left to offer when the hope has spilled out; when I stand in the gap, powerless and spent? When the drips are as high as they can go and there is no more room on the ventilator settings and I stand at the bedside with the loneliness swashing over me, wondering if someone else would do something different, would think of something else?

I glance up to see Lindsey and her husband in the doorway. He pushes the wheelchair across the room and she rises, stooped, slowly straightening up as the ragged tissues in her abdomen elongate. He stands off to the side, says nothing—I never know his name.

I lower the incubator a little for Lindsey and she has eyes only for Ava. Lindsey hasn't changed since I last saw her, her brown hair still braided into pigtails, her face still holding the summer's tan. This time I notice three earrings per ear, one at the top rim, the other two on the fleshy lobe. When she looks at me there is softness in her eyes and her smile is unguarded. I wonder about denial, misunderstanding, optimism, my own ability to communicate. Her countenance remains unchanged as I speak about having to turn up the blood pressure drips, about how Ava is not getting enough oxygen into her bloodstream, about how the ventilator is working as hard as it can. She seems to look through me and somehow, when she smiles, it makes me think that everything will be okay.

The hours pass, and at three in the morning, Ava's blood pressure slips lower. I start an epinephrine drip and give steroids, then take the stairs up to Lindsey's room. The gibbous moon backlights the pictures on the window and casts the sleeping couple in a milky glow. I think of their toddler at home asleep. I think of my own children in their beds, my wife alone in our bed, and the way that same moon shines out over the pines in our backyard. After they rub sleep from their eyes and prop themselves up on their elbows, I tell them—the blood pressure medicine is dosed as high as it can go, the ventilator is doing all it can, the steroids are infusing. All we can do is wait. I look at Ava's mother, who in this moment doesn't need my sympathy or empathy or understanding. She needs me to save her baby. She murmurs acknowledgement, says she will be down in an hour, and I retreat from the room with a hollowness in my marrow.

Ava is alive in the morning. I go home to sleep and have shallow, ambiguous dreams that carry a sense of lightness. When I wake up, I brew coffee, being generous with the scoops, and somehow, I know deep down that the night is behind us and that today Ava rallied. I am content and warm with the feeling of it.

I sit at the kitchen table with the laptop open and the medical record pulled up and hear the sounds of my children playing on the driveway. A cardinal rests on the crepe myrtle, cocks his head, then flies out over the lawn. I read that two hours and thirty-five minutes after I left the hospital the capillaries in Ava's lungs burst and blood filled her air sacs and she drowned. Four minutes later she was dead. The lines unfold and I think about how I don't want to know this—not now, as if not knowing makes it untrue. I think of Lindsey's husband moving up and down the elevator, hauling away five weeks of clothes and books and toiletries. I think of him carefully un-taping the pictures from the window.

The next day I pick my daughter up from Sunday school, passing the twos and threes classroom. A girl sets a doll into a stroller, a boy pushes a fire truck, and another girl sits coloring at a low bench. I look in on their small world, see the girl guide the stroller towards me. I blink and she is Ava. The parents are lining up, pressing stickers to paper, signing the children out, gathering artwork. I blink again and the girl is no longer Ava, just a fleeting image of who Ava might have become. I pass that door, move onto the next, and my daughter runs to me. I scoop her up, kiss her forehead, tuck a Styrofoam cup with eyes and a nose glued to it under my arm, and exit into a throng of people.

A week later I walk under a canopy of green with the dappled shade on the pathway. A lizard startles me as it accelerates through the foliage, a bird sings a song that reminds me of the New Zealand tui of my childhood, and the sound of the wind through the trees reminds me of those tall trees on my college campus, perched on low-slung mountains overlooking the Pacific. Here the earth is rich like coffee grounds, dragonflies drone, and the light is full, clear, and fresh like there never was a night and I feel that I am missing something, something I have yet to comprehend. But all I can think of is the father un-taping the pictures from the window.

Journey of Faith

By necessity, in my earlier years of working as a doctor I focused on the immediate tasks and needs in front of me, on the technical aspects and the objective medicine. But over time my capacity to look beyond momentary needs increased, and both the backgrounds and experiences of families navigating the intensive care unit came more fully into view. Over weeks and months, details of their lives emerged, the pieces of their story coalesced, and I became woven into the fabric of their lives as they became a part of mine.

I met Brian and Esther in the operating room late one night, where we were strangers thrust together in one of life's most intimate moments. This is their story.

Several years before I met them, they moved from Nairobi, Kenya to North Carolina.

Brian found work in mechanical engineering, Esther at a senior center. Fourteen years of marriage, eleven years of praying for a baby, three miscarriages. Then one day an egg caught in the tunnel of her right fallopian tube and it seemed a suitable place to grow, dark and warm and bathed in nutrients. But it was a trap. Soon the egg pushed against the tunnel walls, constricted and hemmed in. The pain in her side exploded in white flames, sucking in on itself before bursting again. Esther lost that fallopian tube and most of her hope. She tried to imagine a life without children and saw empty months stretching into years, season by season; her prayers ascended from brokenness.

Esther carried trays of food to elderly residents: pureed lunch meat, soft potatoes, and lukewarm paper cups of coffee. The wide-open hall smelled of bleach and stale urine and the soft, somber sadness of expired vitality. A TV played old black-and-white movies, and outside the wind pulled at the leaves. That day, in the retirement home, a tiny, lone egg nuzzled into Esther's uterine wall.

The days stretched out, lengthened with worry. She longed for home with the dust and commotion and smell of diesel fuel; she longed for girl-hood, when the world was as big as her street and she moved about encased in a love she never questioned or knew to identify. Now she carried the egg longer than any other. She and Brian wondered if they could allow them-selves to pull the baby book from the shelf where it sat partially hidden between a thick text on engineering and a gardening book. After six weeks, the book came out, an admission of hope, and sat on Esther's bedside table where visitors would not see it. But Esther saw it constantly, brushing it when she turned off the alarm clock in the morning, passing it on her way to the bathroom, in the evening when she changed from her work clothes. When she woke in the night, her hand strayed to the dog-eared cover and felt the springy thickness of the book—a million promises, a million chang-es occurring invisibly every day.

The days slid by and their fetus grew, cells multiplying, organs de-veloping, a constant progression. Unconsciously, Esther kneaded her belly, fingers running down the declivity, feeling the firmness of that slight bulge, feeling the life forming under the tips of her fingers. Her clothes fell over the bulge and she walked with her secret, bubbling within. She wanted to shout it out. One afternoon, she helped Mr. Brigham into a cardigan and slippers. He smelled of talc and called Esther by his daughter's name. No one came to visit him anymore, his family frozen in pictures that seemed to hold no meaning for him. Esther told him, hearing herself saying the words, that she was pregnant, and he grinned a dentured smile, mumbling, the secret already safely lost.

The pressure in her uterus steadily grew like swollen water behind a dam. By eleven weeks her cervix tired and stretched. Reinforcing stitches were threaded through the muscle. Once again, the days grew long in the waiting. She woke up each morning, still pregnant.

At seventeen weeks, Esther was admitted to the hospital on bed rest. That night, with her legs propped up in a mechanical hospital bed, she read how her baby's skeleton was changing from soft cartilage to bone, that the umbilical cord was growing stronger and thicker, that her baby now weighed about as much as a turnip.

Her room on the antenatal ward was stark and empty, the walls an indistinct white. A gap in the window shade let in a sliver of streetlight and muffled sounds tracked through the heating duct. Directly across from the bed, a whiteboard with the names of her doctor and nurse was attached to the wall—the names never changed. She wanted to update it each shift but dared not move. They told her the baby had no chance of survival if she delivered in the next six weeks.

Nameless, shapeless days shifted on. The room so quiet, and days lethargic with the flipping of TV channels: network news, sitcom reruns, and detective shows. She paged through magazines full of glowing, glossy women with perfect skin and hair: how to lose twenty pounds in two weeks, the trick to a perfect complexion. She quickly knew all the nurses by name and when they came into the room she gushed with thankfulness and asked about their families. Each day seemed an hour longer than the day preceding it and Esther found herself looking at the clock incessantly, waiting for Brian to finish work. Those evenings he sat on the edge of the bed and they ate dinner together. It was almost as if they were dating again, with their shyness when the nurses came in and him leaving in the late night. Brian moored her to some sense of herself.

It was late summer, the air still warm, holding the heaviness into the evening. In my small office, I microwaved leftovers for dinner and leafed through a medical journal. The blinds only came down three quarters of the way and outside I could see the dull orange of the parking lot, the light reflecting off scattered cars. One floor below, women lay in bed, anticipating the contractions and pain of labor. Over my desk, the thin fluorescent light bulb hummed, the office filled with the smell of microwaved coconut lentils and rice. I spooned food into my mouth, and it was then that Esther's cervix gave way. She was twenty-four weeks pregnant: one week past the nebulous line of viability but still dangerously early. The baby was breech, the head up under Esther's diaphragm and one foot protruding through the open cervix—it would be too hazardous to attempt a vaginal delivery.

As I slipped on a surgical cap and tied the mask strings behind my head, I saw Brian sitting alone in the hallway outside the operating room, waiting while they prepared his wife for surgery. He wore a white disposable jumpsuit over his clothes, a puffy blue bouffant hat, and a mask. His face was quiet and kind, eyes white against the darkness of his skin. I hastily introduced myself; his handshake was firm and heavy as I felt him transfer his protective role to me, for that moment.

Part Two: Young Attending

Twenty minutes after the call, Faith was pulled from the open cavity of her mother's abdomen, limp and blue and cradled impossibly in the obstetrician's hands. When she was laid on the warmer, her heart slowed. The smell of cauterized flesh drifted across the room and the hot bulb of the warmer irradiated my scalp. Behind me, the obstetrician tied down bleeding vessels, placing thick rail-track sutures across Esther's swollen uterus. The tiny metal blade of the laryngoscope filled Faith's mouth, her jaw pliant as soft cartilage. Everything hinged on the little clear breathing tube angling up, twisting and floating through the swollen miniature vocal cords. I held my breath as the tube bumped up against the cords and slid. There was no guarantee that I would be able to get the breathing tube in place; no matter how many times I am successful, the fear is always there that one day it will prove impossible.

That night the tube went beautifully; her sluggish heart rate, buoyed by the oxygen, increased. I waved to Brian and he came carefully in his disposable shoe covers past the instrument table to stand gazing down at his daughter: parchment-paper skin and blue veins meandering like latticework under downy black hair. Eyelids fused, each rib visible with her belly mushrooming out and arms splotched with mulberry bruises. His daughter: twice the weight of his heart, the weight of a loaf of bread or can of soup, splayed out a little less than the length of his shoe. He stood suspended in the moment while the motion of the city slackened and the night drifted deeper.

Faith, in a clear transport incubator, was wheeled over to her mother, her body strapped to the cross of the operating room table. The angle was awkward, with the incubator two feet higher than the table, the blankets bundled and obscuring Esther's view. On the other side of the drape the suction gurgled, pulling red froth into the canister. Nausea gushed up and over Esther and she retched into a plastic container. Her eyes swam. In the cool of the operating room with the monitor softly beeping, she memorized her baby. We lingered and then pulled away, Brian trailing and my eyes on the saturation monitor; past the viewport of the waiting room, feeling the lurch of the elevator as we moved Faith toward her new home.

Inside the room a small team gathered around an illuminated incubator: nurses in matching azure scrubs, a respiratory therapist twisting gas lines into the back of the ventilator, and a nurse practitioner with pink sneakers waiting to put orders into the computer. The roof of the incubator was raised, with steady heat melting down onto crisp white sheets pulled tight over a thin mattress. At eye level, to the left of the incubator, blinked tandem computer screen monitors; to the right a ventilator, robotic and massive, the tubing alone thicker than Faith's arm. All around on the floor, behind the equipment, spilled tangles of wires and hoses, all anchored to the wall behind. From the base of the incubator, a central line cart jutted into the room. Faith was lifted into the middle of the crowded machinery. I looked at her, thinking of all that could go wrong, and the weight of responsibility surged over me again. Her brain with its fine strands of blood vessels, burrowed deep and liable to rupture; her eyes with immature vessels prone to disorder; her lungs with air spiraling and echoing through the tunnels, erupting into debris-filled soggy lung sacs; her abdomen with fifty inches of poorly vascularized small intestine as delicate as wet paper. I was seeing all that could go wrong, that had, in others, gone wrong, and hoping that for Faith it would not.

Brian was thirty-six, two years older than Esther. He was gentle, soft-spoken and looked at others with sure, steady eyes, seeing the good in them. I noticed later his kindness to Esther and the way he complemented her way of seeing the good in others: his was a quiet knowing, hers more voracious and active. We stood there with the nurses bustling about, Esther still in surgery and Faith before us. I described to Brian how Faith was doing, and when he smiled at her it was lopsided, with more teeth visible on the left.

In the recovery room, a nasal cannula looped from Esther's ears and her breathing was soft and sleepy. When we entered the room, her eyelids fluttered and opened, and I wondered if she recognized me now that my hat and mask were removed. She smiled a drowsy smile and I softly shook her tethered hand, the back sealed in clear tape, flashes of dried blood flanking the IV. Brian held the tips of her fingers while my words skidded around, telling the good points—"She is stable on the ventilator and not needing too much oxygen"—only to qualify them with, "but being born so early, she is at high risk for complications." The impossible dance of allowing for hope but being honest and offering some preparation for the likely bad news to come.

Soon afterwards I stood at Faith's bedside. The numbers on the monitor flashed red as her blood pressure slipped and the machine emitted monotone beeps. I was tired. Around us I could feel the night thick with darkness. Faith barely moved, her skin ashen, the life in her ragged. The medicine dripped in and her blood pressure continued to sink. I paced the hallway, increasing the dose every few minutes until the fluid ran at its maximum rate. When I called the pharmacist to order the second medication, my voice betrayed urgency and soon a pharmacy technician in bright red scrubs passed through the double doors and handed off a foil-wrapped bag like a baton. By four in the morning, Faith's blood pressure was stable. Around the tiny baby were vials of antibiotics; clear bags on IV poles, their thin tubing running through the bowels of rowed pumps; two ventilators working in tandem, brilliant blue light beaming down—a cockpit of monitors, suction dials, ventilator knobs, and buttons.

Her parents understood the odds. They knew, after the eleven years of waiting, the seven weeks of bed rest, the truncated six-month pregnancy, that the chances would not be good. I felt guilty that I could make no promises, but they would not accept my guilt, offering only thanks. Gratitude radiating in front of them, trailing behind, Esther with her head dancing sideways and her effusive smile. Even later, when Faith was stalled on the ventilator, steroids coursing through her body to dampen down the inflammation in the hope of somehow freeing her from the machine, Esther asked about everyone else.

After three days Esther was discharged from the hospital. I imagined her and Brian going home together that first time, down the same streets, Brian driving, Esther gazing out the window, her reflection flashing back as the sun sprung through gaps in the trees. I pictured them walking through their front door, now parents and yet, just as when she was pregnant, still unsure whether they would emerge from the wreckage with a baby. The phone ringer on high and wondering every time the phone rang if it was the hospital. The soreness in the cesarean scars a constant reminder of her tiny baby on the ventilator. The house was no quieter than before Faith, yet her absence inhabited every space. Without meaning to, they saw her in each room: nursing on the couch, grasping little fistfuls of Cheerios in the kitchen, crawling the length of the hallway. Brian couldn't bring himself to put together the crib, hidden in its box and covered with an old blanket in the downstairs closet. That blanket took on significance, the bulge underneath it embodying their life.

Brian went back to work. As I rushed to get ready each morning I thought of Brian and Esther starting their own day, their mornings alive with the patter of coffee in the carafe, steam billowing out the top of the shower, shaving at the sink. Then Brian pulling the door shut and walking down the front path under a canopy of leaves. I imagined Esther attempting to move purposefully about the desperately silent house, tidying small messes, running a load of laundry. Motherhood engulfing her and transforming her being.

Late each morning, Esther drove to the hospital. There was the familiar hiss of the double front sliding doors, the lurch of the faux-wood-paneled elevator, the heavy click of the NICU doors, the warm water and medicated soap at the porcelain sink, and then three pods down the hallway, her baby.

Esther and Brian attended rounds at the bedside each morning and heard, "Her weight today is 620 grams up twenty from prior; she's on the Jet with a rate of 420, PIP 24, PEEP 6, no back up, FiO2 35 percent. Fluids are at 140 mL/kg/day with TPN and intralipids and she's NPO. She's on day one of ibuprofen for a PDA. This morning she had a white count of 11, crit 26, platelets 73, and has been given both PRBCs and platelets. On day four of seven of amp / gent. Sodium 133, potassium 4.3, chloride 105, bicarb 16, BUN 43, creatinine 1.12, glucose 113, and calcium 8.9. UAC at T6 and UVC at T9. Cranial ultrasound to rule out IVH scheduled for Friday." Nothing in English. Esther and Brian looked at the faces in the circle to discern if the words were good or bad, wanting to nod in acknowledgement, to add something helpful.

At first, Faith's nutrition came from yellow IV bags and milky fat syringes, her mouth swabbed with her mother's colostrum. Then after a week, her mother's milk dripped into her stomach, a feeding pump counting out the time. Milliliters at first, then more each day, an entire day's feeding the equivalent of two shots. Often Esther would round the corner to see a tiny red bag hanging from the IV pole. Burgundy blood squeezed from the fatty marrow of a college student, firefighter, or grandmother, each drop migrating to a new labyrinth of dark tunnels, molecular Sherpas bearing oxygen on their backs.

On the seventh day an ultrasound beam gently probed the soft spots, scanning between Faith's cranial bones. On the monitor, pixelated black-and-white grains revealed an otherworldly terrain of submerged caverns and grottos, mountain ridges and deep valleys. The fluid-filled ventricles were homogeneously dark—there was no bleeding in her brain.

For the first part of her hospitalization the ventilator seemed to define her. The tubes running from the torso of the machine anchored Faith to the bed, a constant reminder that she might not make it home. Over the weeks there was forward progress as the ventilator settings were turned down and she seemed to gain strength.

Then one morning, Esther came in to find that the oxygen had been turned up and the ventilator was working harder than ever before. A slimy adherent bacterium trailed down the breathing tube and swarmed Faith's lungs. All gains were erased. Once again, antibiotics trawled her vessels as yellow crept onto the ends of the leaves outside, the air growing lighter, the sun diffuse.

After what seemed an eternity, one month after her birth, the ventilator was turned off. A CPAP machine took its place, then a nasal cannula. At two months her parents saw her face with only the feeding tube: plump cheeks, delicate red lips.

Each gain seemed to be mitigated by a loss, one hurdle crossed only to be followed by another. There was the surge of hope as her oxygen was turned down; the surge of despair as she needed another blood transfusion. Even simple things such as being fed took on mammoth proportions. Towards the end of her tube feeds milk oozed from her mouth and her oxygen saturations fell, her heart rate following. Often, she swallowed and everything righted itself; other times, they both continued falling and her nurse would gently shake her, suction her mouth, and occasionally blow oxygen under her nose. Each day a halting step; the finish line a mirage.

Outside, the late fall had turned from the brilliance of reds and yellows to threadbare trees. Frost glazed the windows in the morning, bitter winds scuttled across the parking lot, and steam curled into the air from the heating exhaust vents. Each morning, with a recliner tipped back, Esther slipped Faith and her tangle of wires down the front of her shirt, Faith's skin against her own, her heartbeat drubbing under Faith's ear, the familiar scent of Esther's skin washing over her baby like rain falling on one's homeland.

After eleven weeks Faith took her first feed from a bottle. The nipple slipped in her mouth and surprised, she did nothing, her face still and motionless while her feeding therapist coaxed the nipple over her pink lip. Soft and comfortable and warm. Milk dripped out and she gagged, her heart rate sliding. That was enough for the first day. Each day was similar. It seemed hopeless. I assured Esther and Brian that she would get it—just give it time. After one week she was able to suck weakly and when I saw her feed I silently chanted *suck, swallow, breathe*, but instead she sucked and breathed at the same time, then tried to swallow. For a preterm baby, feeding is like trying to take the SAT while running upstairs. Yet over the weeks her feeding volumes increased, going from just a few milliliters to whole syringes. Her heart rate remained labile, plunging out of the blue during sleep, plunging during feeds. She would have died if not for the constant presence of her nurses.

Each day I walked the hallway of the NICU with the heaviness that comes of brokenness, much of which cannot be repaired: babies with strokes, brain damage from difficult deliveries, bloodstream infections, varying extremes of prematurity, babies withdrawing from their mothers' drugs. The subversive voice in my head was wondering if someone else would do a better job with these babies. Was I missing something? Many days parents were upset, and their grief turned outward toward me, the person who couldn't make it all better and who couldn't predict the future. And those days I would see Esther and Brian walking down the hallway towards me, smiles visible before anything else, Esther's open arms offering a hug of joy and gratitude. That day-in, day-out consistency of hope was unattached to how Faith was doing clinically; it was a vibrant, living peace and joy. People wondered what its source was. I knew—I had seen it in others and recognized it—a deep, unrelenting faith in a good God.

Brian and Esther's joy challenged my bewilderment about the pain I saw around me and my questioning of God's goodness. I saw in them something I longed for.

One night around that time, I attended an evening gathering of men from church, eight of us squeezed onto couches and chairs in a living room. I carried with me a smiling veneer but underneath I was reluctant and hostile and cynical. Yet despite my misgivings, I was drawn by a thirst for the kind of peace and joy I saw in Brian and Esther.

We studied a book about the goodness of God. The pages felt like a provocation, and I argued each point. Memories strobed before me: a bald teenage girl with a red bandana, children with the yellow-gray pallor of sepsis, listening to a baby's chest and my own thick voice telling the parents there was no heartbeat. My paradigm collided with that of our host, but he overflowed with love and a joyful eagerness that I couldn't deny. He revealed a God who could redeem anything but who did not cause the underlying tragedy. The concepts were not new to me, just lost and scattered and torn, dragged through the mud and sullied beyond recognition.

That night I began to shed the fallacy that everything that happens is the will of God—a fallacy that, when carried to its conclusion, makes God the author of childhood cancer and sepsis and any other number of atrocities. Over the following weeks something changed in me. I felt the fight leave me, felt the residue of the years strip away and had the sensation of coming back to a place I'd been gone from for some time, a place familiar and certain. I was overcome by a feeling of returning.

Back in the hospital, I stood over Faith's bed a changed man. And she was changing too, her cheeks now full and round, her body filling in the newborn onesies. Beneath downy hair and soft tectonic plates of bone, neurons amassed, the cortex of her brain folding into aqueous valleys. Over three months the size of her brain had increased 400 percent. And yet it seemed that things could never all come together for her. She had reached her due date and her lungs were still heavy with fluid, her air sacs underdeveloped. Her breathing became rapid with feeding. Milk escaped from the side of her mouth and still her heart rate plunged unexpectedly.

In the open crib with her pink newborn clothes and a receiving blanket swaddling her, she looked as though she could go home that day. Only the feeding tube gave her away. When her parents held her, she was full and robust in their arms and I thought of that first month when they held her against their bare chests, with the knot of wires and tubes, the monitors screeching, her body impossibly fragile and weightless, her dry, thin skin and the deep creases across her brow giving her an old, wise face.

As quickly as it started, it ended. Faith sucked contentedly at her bottle or at the breast, her heartbeat steady. A diuretic medicine was squirted into a nippleful of milk twice a day and bailed out her lungs enough that she could breathe comfortably. I talked about her at home, and my children made congratulation cards for her out of folded construction paper and crayons. Across the dinner table, strands of hair fell over my wife's cheeks, her gaze quiet and deep. She had been with me from the start, through each stage of my journey. I thought of her yelling at the rowdy teenagers who were keeping us awake the night before my medical school boards, the countless nights she spent alone with me away at the hospital, the missed social events, and of hauling her across the country for my medical training. I thought of the stress I carry into the house after work and of the blessing of coming home to her—my wife with kind greenstone eyes, my bedrock and joy.

Over the last several days before she went home, Faith's parents snapped pictures of the staff holding her. In those pictures the nurses look into the lens with proud eyes and hold her close, as if she were their own. In my picture, Faith wears a frilled hat and a matching jumpsuit, all white and pink, and looks with an unfocused gaze to the left of the camera. I can see the pride in my own eyes, and relief, and an unguarded smile.

Three years later I saw Faith's parents again in the operating room. Esther lay on the table, a blue drape ascending from her chest, with the obstetricians standing on either side of her, the scalpel sliding down again and again until clear fluid burst out and the cavity was flooded. She was awake, her makeup strangely out of place with the steel instruments and swimming red on the other side of the drape. Brian sat on a stool by her head and they wore the same familiar, broad, overflowing smiles. Even with her abdomen spliced open and her baby almost born, she asked how I was doing. That morning a healthy, full-term daughter was born. The overhead lights reflected off the clear sheen of her, eyes scrunched tight and lungs open wide. When they held her, it seemed strange—I had only ever seen them hold Faith. After all our history, I was with them for just a short time that morning.

Six months after that moment I sat in a wooden pew under a vaulted ceiling, stained glass narratives suffusing the room in ethereal light. Far above me to the right, Jesus walked on water, calm and sure. Parents readied their cameras, shifting eagerly; grandparents sat captivated by the bounce of perfect curls and the shine of little white teeth. On the stage the preschoolers shifted and bobbed in reds and greens. One little girl with shoulder-length brown hair called out a hello to Grandpa. The children sang unevenly and off-key, some with zealous gusto, others looking tepidly into the crowd. I gazed at my daughter, standing with hands clasped in front of her tall, slender frame, her face still round with baby fullness, fine straight hair, deep walnut eyes and thin red lips. Next to me sat my wife and parents and I felt the rush of time sweeping us up, with my last baby singing on the stage, growing older before my eyes. The class filed out and the next took their place. I could see Faith in the front row towards the right, her voice swallowed in the chorus. Strange to think I saw her before her mother ever did, before her father. I watched her singing; her earnest face swept me in wonder.

The children swayed and sang, and parents crouched in the aisles, pointing phones towards the stage. Esther turned from several pews in front of me and our eyes met. We smiled, our hearts full with the shared dreams of parents and a flooding gratitude.

Becoming

Withdrawal

S ome transitions are marked by a day on the calendar or a change
in location: the last day of medical training, the flight home from
a war, or the move from one company to another. Others are more nu-
anced, only seen in retrospect. As the years passed and the distance from
my years of training increased, the practice hired new doctors and I was
no longer the new guy. My children grew and my marriage deepened. I
presume there are some jobs that become easier with time, but medicine
is not one of them.

One day around mid-morning, a nurse called me from the mother-
baby floor to request an evaluation for a three-day-old boy. Outside the
room and even down the hall, you could hear his shrill cry. The sound was
incessant, breaking only long enough for him to gasp for breath then wail
again. He was red-faced, scratch marks ran down his cheeks, his arms and
legs quivered, and he turned his head back and forth, flailing inside his
plastic box of a crib.

In the bed his mother snored, her head lolled to one side, the sheets
twisted over her waist, the air thick with the smell of stale tobacco and
sweat.

"Hi, Ms. Wilson, I'm Dr. Rattray from the NICU," I said loudly.

She startled, her eyes glazed over, and her head fell back into the cavity
of the pillow.

"Ms. Wilson—I came to check on your baby."

Once again, Nikki Wilson startled, this time pulling herself into a
sitting position. She rubbed her eyes, squinted at me, and reached out to
pat her baby's chest. Her hair was black and disheveled. Dollops of dis-
coloration patched her cheeks and a fading tattoo stretched along her left

forearm. Her sallow, sleepy face carried a flatness; she looked world-weary, as if anything good or true had either been lost or was only ever a mirage. Every minute her eyelids crawled down until she jerked them back up seconds later. I took in her screaming baby, the ineffective patting of his chest, the hollowness of her cheeks, and wondered how she got here. How tiny molecules like snowflakes—carbon, oxygen, nitrogen stitched together in pentamers, hexagons, carbon appendages jutting like docks—could hold such sway over someone. Every year these same molecules tumble through the bloodstreams of millions of people in the United States. Every year babies float in wombs, muffled soundwaves rippling through the fluid, light filtering into the gloaming, the lifelines of the umbilical cords bringing glucose, oxygen, protein, fat, carbohydrates, calcium, and drug metabolites.

Why take the oxycodone at the party, why try a roommate's pain pills? I hear so many different stories. I met a woman who became dependent on opioids after back surgery for scoliosis. Another started by taking oxycodone at a party and then switched to heroin because it was cheaper, and another started using heroin to numb the pain after her toddler drowned. What about the first time for Nikki? Was it a sense of hopelessness that blanketed her in pain? Perhaps something inside her just slipped, like a door not quite latched, and with a quick toss of her head, the pill traversed her esophagus, plunged into the acidity of her stomach, and rapidly dissolved. Did the pill, like a kaleidoscope, cause a different world to float before her eyes? Surely Nikki couldn't have thought of the future when she took that first hit. The trap had sprung.

I wonder what it feels like when the chemicals tumble through the bloodstream. Does it feel like floating, like being removed from it all, emotions disconnected and cocooned in lamb's wool? Does it feel like those rare moments when every detail is noticed and heightened? A breathy first kiss, a surfer dropping into a wave, the blurring of time across the wall of water, a prayer that pulls heaven to earth, the soft smell of a newborn's skin? Is it a melting away of the chattering voice in one's head, a dissolving of all worries and fears, a slight slowing of the heart rate and a dip in the blood pressure? Could it be that the molecules bring forgiveness for all shortcomings? Or perhaps they simply numb us to the point where there is no need for forgiveness. In that unearned peace, the future is unimportant.

I want to understand. I want to empathize.

A week before my daughter was born, I pulled shrubs from the front planter next to the mailbox. Later that day my hands and lower arms erupted: red, weepy, swollen and so itchy I wanted to scrape the skin off. The dermatologist prescribed prednisone tablets and steroid cream. The prednisone washed away my fatigue. Instead of my usual afternoon lull in energy I was focused and ready to take on anything, and in the evenings, I worked into the night with energy to spare. A week later, when it came time to start the taper off the prednisone, I realized I would miss that energy boost. It reminded me of a fellow medical student I met during a neurosurgery rotation. We formed an immediate friendship. We changed into scrubs together at four in the morning, raided the cracker stash behind the nurse's station when hypoglycemia set in, and stood in the same ORs for nine-hour surgeries. One day he told me that he took cocaine during finals to stay awake and cram—most of his friends did. He said it gave him energy, kept him alert and focused. At the end of the rotation, he stole my neurosurgery textbook and went back to Florida.

Years later my wife and I moved into a new house. We slept the first night on blow-up mattresses in the kitchen nook with the moving truck expected the next day. The next morning, I realized that I didn't have a coffee maker. As the morning wore on, a band ratcheted around my head and I became nauseated. As I sat on the front step waiting for the moving truck, my body cried out for caffeine. This must be what drug addiction is—physical pain until the desired molecules float through the bloodstream, satiating the angry receptors.

I placed a stethoscope on the baby's chest but couldn't hear over his screams. His mouth rooted frantically for my gloved finger and he sucked hard on my knuckle. Red linear scratches crossed his cheeks. He trembled and his arms and legs wound tight into flexion, pulled in hard against his body.

"What's his name?" I asked.

"Kamryn with a 'K,'" she said.

"That's a great name. Well, as you know, his withdrawal scores have been really high," I said.

She shook her head. "He just started crying. He's hungry."

I picked up the screaming baby and handed him to her. She held him close, forcing a bottle into his mouth, and he tried to suck but couldn't co-ordinate the motion and instead threw his face back and forth and wailed.

"His scores over the past day have been high, not just when he's hungry. We worry about babies going through withdrawal because they can have seizures and get sick."

"He's not withdrawing bad—he would be okay, but the nurses keep waking him up. They keep giving him high scores because they know I took Percocet. I see how they look at me."

"I'm sorry you feel that way. We just want to make sure that we're taking good care of him. Can you tell me a little bit about your pregnancy?"

"Well, it was fine really except that I had a lot of pain in my back and legs."

"Do you know what the pain was from?"

"They said it was sciatica from the baby pressing on me."

"And what medicines did you take during the pregnancy?"

"Just my prenatal vitamins and Percocet. My grandmother had some leftover Percocet, so she helped me out and gave me some. The doctors wouldn't help me so that's all I could do."

"Had you used anything before you were pregnant?"

"Yeah, I got in with the wrong crowd after high school. I smoked marijuana and took oxy. But I stopped before the pregnancy—I can stop that whenever I want. I just took Percocet during pregnancy for my back. My grandma feels really bad now, she says she shouldn't have given me her pills, but she saw how much pain I was in."

She didn't tell me the whole story. Her drug tests during pregnancy showed metabolites of opioids, benzodiazepines, cocaine, and amphetamines. I knew from a nursing note that Nikki had taken ecstasy the day after her C-section. The chemical milieu amazed me, a wild rollercoaster of central nervous system depressants and stimulants.

I thought of Nikki pregnant, of how the cravings and necessity of the drugs took over and despite the rounded belly, the fluttering and tumbling within her, her body navigated towards the bottle or Ziploc bag and she opened the lid, extracted one or two pills, and propelled them down her throat. Of how she divided a portion of white powder, rolled a piece of paper, and snorted hard. When I stood in the room, I felt a heaviness, a hopelessness. I stood before a woman who lived as a slave, in bondage to chemicals that she knew would damage her baby, would lead to child protective services placing him with another family; chemicals to which she would give away her body and last shreds of dignity.

I knew it could happen to anyone. One night, years ago, I sat with a small group of men. Across from me was David, a soft-spoken, gentle man who greeted everyone with a hug. That night he told a story. He came home with his wife one evening and found his adult son on their couch, barely breathing and unresponsive. I imagined the red lights of the ambulance spinning off the front walls of the house, the paramedics heaving David's son onto the stretcher, the legs collapsing up as they slid him into the back of the ambulance. I couldn't help but ask myself, *If David couldn't protect his son from an overdose, then how can I protect my own children?* Perhaps we can rationalize it when it happens to people who have suffered abuse or neglect or have untreated mental illness, but what about when it happens to our children, whom we have loved and cared for and provided for? Unlike a broken bone, addiction is invisible and unquantifiable.

Nikki kept trying to give Kamryn the bottle. He sucked vigorously for a second, collapsing the nipple, then threw his head to the side, milk dribbling down the corner of his mouth. She tried again and again, while he shrieked and swatted the bottle with a free hand.

"What will you treat him with?" she asked me over his cries.

"Morphine."

"No, not morphine. Can't you use Tylenol?"

"No, we can't use Tylenol. We have to match up what we treat him with to what he was getting in the womb, an opioid to treat opioid withdrawal."

"Do you really have to give him that? I don't want him to get morphine. It's not good for him."

Anger swept over me. Her baby was too frantic to feed. He was jittery, trembling and thrashing. Surely Nikki knew what it was like to go through withdrawal—the sweating, sleeplessness, muscle aches, anxiety, diarrhea, abdominal cramps, nausea, and vomiting—and she would never consider treating her own withdrawal with Tylenol. Yet here she was asking me to let her son go through withdrawal without adequate treatment.

I took a deep breath and looked out the window. She must have known all along that child services would take him just as they had taken her two girls. And yet somehow, she seemed hopeful that this time it would be different. That with this new baby she would have a clean start. She seemed to see him though a different lens. She didn't see the exaggerated tremble of his arms and legs; she didn't hear the high-pitched, frantic cry or notice the loose watery stools that seeped through the diaper. When she held him, she didn't seem to feel the tightness coiled in his body, the flexing arms and legs, or see the pale latticework of skin across his chest, the over-vigorous suck that collapsed the nipple of the bottle. And to me it seemed that when she saw his wrinkled forehead, he appeared wise, as though he knew all that she didn't, and when she looked into his eyes and he blinked up at her, she saw an ocean of forgiveness.

"Yes, we have to give him morphine. He's withdrawing really badly. Think about how it feels when you've weaned off something. He's going through the same thing. When he was born it was like going cold turkey."

"I just don't want him to have to get treated."

"I know, it's tough. But we'll start at the lowest dose we can and wean him off as fast as he lets us."

She knew that when she let him be taken from her arms, when Kamryn left her room, that she might never have him again. Already the cogs were turning, calls were being made. Nikki was being investigated. When they combed through her chart the pieces would come together and a foster family would be called. Perhaps she imagined the family that would take him. A young couple with a ranch-style two-bedroom and flowering pear trees in the front yard. Or perhaps a family with older children, even teenagers, with a little white picket fence and a tire swing in the front yard. Surely the thought made her drown. Her eyes flared and she pulled herself up in bed and I felt her anger, but then she let her eyelids droop and a mask fell over her face. Once more I could see the flatness in her as she let the stream of the world take her.

I left her room hating myself, broken again by something I had done so many times before. It made me angry because I knew I was doing the right thing. Her baby was inconsolable, trembling; he couldn't feed and was close to seizing. Yet I walked away crushed and bewildered. It happens every time. I walked down the hallway, past a watercolor painting of a young mother standing on a beach with a girl. They hold hands and the girl looks up at her mother, her face radiating wonder and trust and adoration. In that moment, I thought of how life often looks so different from that idyllic picture.

I remember twenty years ago, sitting in my car in a hospital parking lot. I crumple into the steering wheel, sobbing so hard I can barely breathe, tears running down the wheel, spilling onto my jeans. I have just seen my niece, hours old and absolutely perfect. She will be going away. I am powerless to stop it. Powerless against wrong timing, wrong circumstances; powerless to stall time while her too-young mother finishes college and becomes an adult ready to raise a child. Instead, her mother makes the ultimate sacrifice and passes her to a family, kind and generous, who will hold her as their own. The world buckles under me, nothing as it was. Now I am on the other side, taking this mother's baby away, and I am still powerless. I know the pain that will collapse over Nikki, again and again.

Emergency Room

I used to think that some memories would fade with time, that I would no longer feel them in my chest or see the images in my mind when I closed my eyes. But one night while lying on my daughter's bed, I realized that is a fallacy. Our lives are built on the bricks of memory. I hold her nine-year-old body close, her sobs vibrating into my chest. I can taste the salt of her tears as they weave from her cheek onto mine. Amongst the shudders of breath, I gather something about Jessica saying that she won't be friends with Hannah if Hannah is friends with Emily. As I hold my daughter close, I see tracks of red under her eyes. Wisps of her blond hair come loose and stick to the corners of my mouth. After a few minutes, her breathing slows and she asks, "Daddy, how come you never cry?"

"Well sweetie, adults don't usually cry as often as kids, but we do cry sometimes."

"Like when? When was the last time you cried?"

"It was a while ago, when you were two."

"What did you cry about? What happened?"

I hesitate, conflicted because I know I can't tell her the story, but I don't know what to say. It seems wrong to lie but I want to protect my daughter from whatever pain and tragedy I can. When her class studied the Holocaust, she cried herself to sleep every night for a week. She reminds me so much of myself as a child. When the Save The Children commercials came on and I saw the barefooted, emaciated toddlers with swollen bellies, their faces blank and studded with flies, I sobbed on my bed, my mother stroking my shoulder. In some ways nothing has changed. The morning news can cripple me: genocide, shootings at churches and mosques, and refugees drowning in the Mediterranean.

I stroke Hannah's hair behind her ears and tell her a version of the truth, "There was a little girl at the hospital and things didn't go the way we wanted them to and it made me sad." Then I change the subject and she lets me plow ahead, leaving the story untold.

But here is what happened.

Shortly after ten in the evening I called my wife from the small community hospital where I was moonlighting to tell her goodnight and that I loved her. There were only eight babies in the special care nursery, all sleeping or feeding. The call room bed looked enticing—I had squeezed this shift in among my frequent overnight calls at the main hospital. Just as I was hanging up with Danielle, the emergency room charge nurse called to say that a toddler was inbound and the ER doctor requested my help.

Moving through the back doors, I came to the central nursing station where the ER doctor, Mike Carter, listened to the crackle of the radio, the siren cutting through the paramedic's raised voice. They were doing CPR. Dr. Carter rolled up his smudged white coat sleeves and ran a hand through his cropped gray hair.

"Thanks for coming down," he said. "We don't get many kids here. I'll take the airway if you can take access."

"Sure," I agreed, trying to sound nonchalant while I shivered under the cool of the air conditioning.

We walked over to the trauma bay and stood, arms crossed, trying to make small talk while the seconds ticked by. The glaring lights overhead turned the bedsheets on the waiting gurney a brilliant white and sheened off the plastic wall cabinets. We chatted about working nights and how busy the ER was that night and soon we heard them coming down the hall, the fast cadence of boots landing on linoleum. They swung into the bay and lifted the girl's limp body onto the gurney; her nightie was cut open down the center and the paramedic's hands rocked hard into her chest.

"She's not breathing, no heart rate. No past medical history. Parents said they checked on her and she wasn't breathing," he huffed.

An ER nurse took over chest compressions while the doctor intubated, and I probed her groin for a femoral vein. Her skin was cool under my fingers and when the blood trickled from the needle it was dark and soupy. I looked at her blonde hair spread out over the pillow and it looked like my daughter's. The nurse paused compressions, the monitor flat and unblinking. "Asystole," said Dr. Carter. "Nothing to shock, resume compressions and epi."

Over my shoulder I could see her parents standing just outside the door, their arms around each other. After twenty minutes of CPR, medications, and fluids, Dr. Carter looked at me and I nodded in agreement. The girl lay on the big gurney with her pudgy arms out, her palms upwards, her face pale; I took a step back, turned, and went into the hallway and told her parents.

I made it out of the ER and to the wide staircase, empty and dim, before I crouched down and cried. Once I started, I couldn't stop. I kept picturing my own daughter lying in her bed, the slight curl of her hair, the way it flowed out over the pillow.

That's the story I can't tell my daughter. And lying on her bed that night feels so near, despite all the years. I wonder if I am the only one who harbors these types of images, while everyone else lets them drift away? For me, certain stories remain, out of the countless others, and that little girl's story is woven into mine.

I hold my daughter close and tell her, "Hannah, there are days when nothing seems to make sense and we feel sort of lost. On those days it's really hard to remember that things will get better. Sometimes it helps to think about something good, maybe a favorite memory or place."

"Like what, Daddy?"

"Let's think. How about that time we sailed out to the island last winter?"

"Yeah, that was fun."

I think back to that day. The NICU was unusually quiet and I drove home early in the throes of a freak warm spell in January. The cherry blossoms, tricked into budding early, stood out against the brown of the leafless trees, glorious and exultant. After the previous months of cold, I felt giddy. My wife and I are planners—we have a paper calendar in the pantry, a white board calendar in the mudroom, and electronic calendars on our phones. But the warmth and sun in the middle of winter drew out a restlessness and as soon as I got home, we cancelled the children's piano lessons and my afternoon meeting and headed for the school to pick up the kids. They each came into the front office with puzzled looks on their faces. "I don't have a doctor's appointment, do I?" asked my son.

"I'll tell you on the way," I told him as I signed him out.

I had an old 1970s sailboat on a trailer at a nearby lake. The boat looked beautiful from far away: nice shapely lines, a white deck, and a baby-blue hull. She was as long as our car and had a little cubby cabin. But on closer inspection the white was more of a faded yellow with tiny cracks and fissures running in every direction, the sail had a small rip in it, and the windows were gray and clouded. The outboard engine started only occasionally, and when it did it would cut out suddenly whenever I was getting blown towards power lines, an oncoming boat, or the shore.

I had driven an hour and a half with my father to buy her the previous summer. It took us longer than expected to get there and the seller had another appointment to get to. I tried to look like I knew what I was doing—knocked on the fiberglass to sound out soft spots, ran my hands over the hull feeling for bulges, and asked probing questions such as, "How does she handle?" I nodded knowingly at the answers and didn't think to ask things like "Does the outboard motor work?" or "Does the boat leak?" I suppose it didn't really matter anyway. I knew I had to have that sailboat. I asked my dad what he thought, and he looked at me apprehensively and shrugged in a way that said: "Not something I would do." So, I said yes and handed over an envelope with a thousand dollars cash in it.

My dad guided me as I reversed the car towards the trailer and I cranked the trailer jack down until the back of my car sagged and the tongue clicked over the hitch. I felt giddy pulling out of that dirt driveway and that feeling helped me ignore the glares of other drivers as I crawled along the freeway with my twenty-one-foot sailboat tied down to a rusted fifty-year-old trailer. Two hours later I pulled into my driveway, white-knuckled and triumphant.

That afternoon my parents and I worked through the tangle of lines and rigging and I spent every evening that next week on the boat in my driveway with my son, scrubbing the inside of the cabin, washing the cushions, tidying the lines, and lying on the thin bunks dreaming of bobbing out at anchor.

After all sorts of mishaps—jammed mainsail sliders, getting blown into the dock, grounding on a sandbar, and the boat almost slipping off the trailer when the strap snapped—we were trying again, driving the half hour to the lake on a bright January day.

After ratcheting the boat into the water I stood on the bow, attaching the foresail with a warm breeze luffing the sail and the sun splintering off the water. That day the sails went up easily, the breeze shaping them into white scoops; to my right, the trees ran up the shore, mostly pine and oak, and there was a lightening of the blue water as the bottom reached out, forming a sandbar when we rounded the point. To my left, a trio of smokestacks steamed behind a ridge of chain-link fence. Every fifteen minutes I dragged a cut-out gallon Clorox container along the inside of the boat, bailing out the silty water.

There was a small island in the center of the lake. Around the periphery, waves slapped against jutted banks and tangles of tree branches overhung the water. We rounded the top part of the island, turned into the wind, and doused the sails. The mast and rigging scraped up against the arms of pines and oaks as we bumped against the island and the children clambered over the side, barefoot in the ankle-deep water. I called for them to wait while I tied a line to a tree trunk and my wife jumped down, following with three pairs of flip-flops.

Here we were only a mile from the shore, but we may as well have been in a remote country. That afternoon we didn't have to cajole Hannah to add and redistribute number patterns or sit in a meeting discussing intractable problems. Two hours ago, I was in the hospital, blinking dry eyes and typing into medical records and now I stood on an island with wet shoes, the pines clattering together, groaning as the wind funneled across the water into them.

We found a sandy cove on the other side and the kids skipped pebbles out into the water, the ripples breaking up the mirrored flawless blue sky; my wife and I stood holding hands, looking at the sky and the water and our children playing, and it felt as though we had been handed a miracle.

Time and distance: new memories shuffle into the seahorse of the hippocampus, some sifting into nothingness, others implanting, the roots burying deep. They become a part of us, change and mold us. This is what I want to tell Hannah—that we will always live with a mosaic of memories, some glinting with light and color, others dark and shadowy. What matters, I think, is how we arrange those pieces; how we let the pieces, azure and lilac and steel and carmine, exist together, each one defining the others.

Reunion

My phone buzzed as a text message came in. It was a video of Brayden standing on his driveway. He held a football in his left hand, wound it up, and sent it flying twelve feet into a catching net. After he sunk the shot, he spun around towards the camera and clapped his hands with glee. His joy made me smile.

The last time I saw Brayden was at the university hospital NICU reunion several years prior. It was the deepest part of summer. By ten in the morning the sun already scorched my scalp and the pavement simmered as I breathed in the humid air. I walked across the parking lot with Jonathan, a friend from training. It was a Saturday, and families pushed babies in strollers and held their children's hands as they thronged around us, everyone making their way across the hot asphalt to the science and nature museum. It seemed like a lifetime ago that I had come here with my own children. I thought of meandering through the outdoor area with my son one day when he was a toddler. We had the day to ourselves. No timetable, no schedule—a magical fall day with the leaves on fire, the smell of damp earth, and my son's little feet taking us wherever he wanted to go. His hair lifted in a wave at the front flowing up over a cowlick, and he wore blue Stride Rites with thick soles. Now, eight years later, I was here for a NICU family reunion held in a tented area to the side of the museum.

We made our way over to the tent, and as I scrawled my name on a sticker someone behind me called out. I turned to see a woman in her mid-thirties in a floral summer dress, a huge smile on her face. She hugged us and looked at me and Jonathan expectantly, waving a preschool-aged boy over. "Look, Brayden, it's the doctors who took care of you!"

Brayden ran over to us, grinning, looking grown-up. He wore a collared shirt and pants, straight blond hair framing a handsome, angular face. His right shoulder was slightly higher than his left. I noticed a gentle bend at his elbow, and the way his right leg drifted inward. I looked once more at his mother and the past came tumbling back. Scattered scenes from his hospitalization flooded my memory: sitting next to the radiant warmer with his parents, the high-frequency ventilator thumping in our ear. A strip of white tape across Brayden's face to hold the breathing tube, that face dwarfed by the earmuffs we placed on him to shield him from the noise of the ventilator. I remembered pulling up a brain MRI to show his parents, pointing out the markings of injury. I remembered his body, so small and bloated, a result of hydrops, a nebulous condition that started in the womb and led to fluid accumulation in his abdomen, around his heart and lungs, and under his skin. I remembered the enveloping bleakness and unrelenting powerlessness I felt. Now, Brayden looked up at us, and I reached down and slapped him five, filled with wonder at his metamorphosis from the labile, fragile baby engulfed in lines and tubes.

Erin absently ran her hand through his hair and pulled him close. Brayden grinned up at us again—he knew he was desperately loved and cherished. Erin thanked us as only a mother could. She thanked us for caring for him, for getting him home. But I couldn't accept it. I felt like an actor, unconvinced of the reality of my own role in Brayden's care. Even now I feel the same way with parents, acquaintances, friends, and family. In her exuberance, my daughter likes to tell people, "My daddy is a doctor," and I think to myself: *Really?* Perhaps these feelings come from all the limitations, all the things I know I cannot fix, like the telltale limp in Brayden's stride. I think of all the other people who cared for him those hours, days, and months; of the nurses who were always with him. What kind of credit do I deserve?

As we talked, Dr. Goldberg, our former program director, joined the group, greeting us like we were children returning home for the holidays. "You're looking thin," he said to me. "Aren't they feeding you over there? Jonathan, haven't you found a Jewish wife yet?"

We stood chatting, Jonathan and I glowing in his light. I thought back to a time during training when I stopped by the office along the back hallway of the NICU. It was the end of a long day and Dr. Goldberg had just come through the door, briefcase in his hand. I asked him his advice about a patient. It wasn't anything particularly serious or pressing, but without a word he put his bag down by the desk and walked to the patient's bedside with me. His investment in us was total, complete.

I remember how it all began, eight years earlier on a hot summer night.

My wife and I stood on the curb, under flickering yellow lights, our four-month-old son in her arms. At our feet lay a stroller, car seat, three oversized bags, and a beagle. Thunder in Dallas; enveloping humidity in Durham. Flights were delayed, and a chain-link barricade blocked off the car rental office. Our fellow passengers quickly dissipated, likely driving home to lights glowing in windows and waiting families. Cigarette smoke seeped down the throughway and the rumble of a truck motor echoed against the concrete walls; beyond the reach of the lights, the dark of our new city stretched out. I hailed a cab, wondering if he would take a baby in a car seat and a dog. A driver, grave and sullen, nodded and I wrestled the car seat onto the back lap belt. It wobbled a little but held tight.

We spent the first night in a nondescript hotel at the side of the freeway. In the early morning light, I looked out over the parking lot at a Waffle House sign and a patch of woods, marveling at how different everything can feel within the same country. F. Scott Fitzgerald wrote, "Most of us have a favorite, a heroic period, in our lives." As I look back on my life, this is that period.

By midmorning we stood on the street looking up at the house we had closed on the week before—Owen on my wife's hip, the birds singing, and the grass uncut. The smell of pear blossoms hung faintly in the air. Up a small rise sat the house, Colonial style white clapboard siding, black shutters, symmetrical windows, and a slight pediment over the front door. Every detail displaced us from the life we had known in California—vines here crawling up the trunks of the trees, the tracts of woods and, especially later during the evenings, the fireflies floating, the heavy drone of cicadas, and the way the humidity held into the night, blanketing the heat. We walked through the house in wonder, having moved from a nine hundred-square-foot condominium to a house three times as large. Looking out of the empty bedrooms onto the backyard studded with gum trees, I pictured where I would build a sandbox. I shook my head with amazement at the trees thick with leaves, the stretch of grass, and, beyond the backyard, a thin tarmac walking path. That afternoon we walked the path, Owen in his stroller, the stream gurgling alongside us, flush with promise. I wore a new

Duke T-shirt, incredulous that they had accepted me into their pediatric residency program. I had the feeling both of years of hard work paying off and of pure, unadulterated luck.

Those were the days when everything was new, our marriage young, and I had never seen a child or baby die. I knew nothing of hospital politics, hospital administration, financial payors, or the threat of litigation. Instead, I saw my baby boy and the green in my wife's eyes. We were blind to the pain our moving away caused our families. We simply felt driven away by the high cost of living in California and the promise of training at Duke.

That first night the sky lit up, flashes like incendiaries out over the oak trees into the horizon. We gazed uncertainly out the window—it wasn't until later that we realized it had been a lightning storm. The house smelled musty and foreign. We slept on a blow-up mattress, our son between us in a sleep positioner, his breath soft and milky, fine creases under his dark eyelashes. The street was pierced by a solitary streetlight illuminating a blossoming pear tree, fading quickly into darkness at the edges. The house opposite was dark; we knew no one. Thunder crumpled the compressed air and the vibrations ran down the doorframes into the carpet. The humid air refused to coalesce into drops and hung hot and heavy.

For all the magic of the house, the construction was shoddy and every effort had been made to save building costs. In the winter I could feel the draft flow in under the window frames, and in the attic, I discovered large swaths of walls that were uninsulated. The first water leak occurred shortly after we moved in. Owen sat in his high chair, gumming cereal puffs. I heard a pop, and then water shot into the kitchen. Grabbing a bucket, I stupidly tried to catch it while yelling to my wife to turn off the water. We didn't know yet that the shut-off was concealed under a built-in wooden box in the hall closet. While water streamed in my face and soaked the floor, Owen sat there grinning and pointing, saying, "Wa, wa. Wa, wa."

Now I stood among families whose babies I had cared for and the feeling was nothing short of surreal. As we stood together for a group picture, I looked over the crowd, everyone smiling, mothers and fathers holding babies and toddlers up for the camera. They had all experienced the same NICU walls, the commotion of delivery, the disquieting noises of machines and monitors. I have only ever experienced the NICU as a physician; those walls are so familiar, yet there is so much I don't know. I have called families in the middle of the night, but never been the one to reach out for the phone in the dark. I have described a treatment plan, but I haven't lived through seeing my own baby on a ventilator. Can that divide be closed? Could I really understand? Would it change the way I approach families? Dare I look out over the crowd and just for this one moment bask in the success?

The feeling of being an imposter remains, no matter what I accomplish, despite publishing journal articles, achieving board certification; despite years of experience. Perhaps it all stems from daily trips to the mailbox when I applied to medical school, the rejection letters piling up, my faith in the future waning. Or perhaps it was the grueling years of medical school training where we were always out of place and in the way, or later during residency, when irate cardiothoracic surgeons yelled at us after we had been awake for thirty hours in the pediatric ICU. Perhaps it's the problems that can't be fixed, the tragic losses that we can't prevent. Maybe it has nothing to do with that. Instead, it may be the mirage of perfection, always shimmering in front of me yet wholly out of reach.

But on that day in the summer sun, standing next to Dr. Goldberg and Jonathan, I let Brayden's mother's smile permeate my imposter skin, let it sink through to meet my own quiet joy.

Kevin

That afternoon, driving home from the reunion, my mind wandered as the miles of freeway slid by. Memories tumbled through me: our house with the white siding and black shutters; the Japanese cherry trees lining the sidewalk outside the hospital; driving home exhausted after those long days during training and pulling into the driveway to see my son standing at the window, a wooden train in each hand. And I thought about Kevin.

The first time I met Kevin was during my second year of pediatric residency training, when he was a brand-new intern. I had entered the residents' workroom at dawn. The workroom was a sort of barracks with banks of computers on one side and a couch with tangled blankets and a conference table on the other. Shoes, jackets, papers, coffee cups, and white coats were strewn around the room. My fingers ran over the laminated code cheat sheet in my white coat pocket, my index finger smoothing down the separating edges. About fifteen people occupied the space: bleary-eyed residents wearing crumpled scrubs, smelling of sour coffee and sweat; crisp medical students in pressed short white coats with thick pocket-edition books and pens neatly lining their pockets; and the subdued oncoming residents.

I scanned the room for Kevin but he saw me first, approaching me with an outstretched hand. "Are we ready to do this, or what?"

Kevin was my intern for the month. This was my first time in the role of senior resident and his first time as an intern on the wards. Just a few months before, he had walked across the stage and graduated from medical school. Our schedule for the month would be simple. We would work together every day from 6 a.m. to 7 p.m., then every third day we would work a thirty-hour call. The days consisted of rounding on the children on the ward, discharging those who were ready to go home, managing problems that arose during the day, and admitting new patients.

It was my job to teach Kevin both the medical and practical aspects of life on the wards. Unfortunately, this included the burden of paperwork. Upon discharge of a patient, we had twenty-four hours to dictate a discharge summary. We were always hopelessly behind, admitting new patients before we had a chance to dictate discharge notes. After the twenty-four hours had elapsed a rubbery, stoic woman in white sneakers, pushing a wire basket, would invade our workroom, fill her basket, and transport the charts down to the bowels of the medical records department. We quickly learned that any attempts to smooth-talk, plead, or threaten would not sway her resolve. The answer was always the same: to finish the dictation, we would have to go down to the records department, fill out a form, and wait for the chart to be located. So instead, we stashed the charts in obscure places as we approached that twenty-four-hour mark. Many times, we went back to retrieve them only to find them missing—she was too good for us. Over time, however, we became more and more resourceful, finding hiding places behind stacks of books, in the microwave, and finally, in the hollow ceiling tiles. These were some of the most important skills I would teach Kevin.

That first day was a frenzy of activity and it was evening before we knew it. We were first to be on call, and looking at the prospect of the night ahead was like looking out across a dark ocean. One by one, the other teams signed out their patients to us and trickled out. As they reported to us Kevin's pager kept going off, the pages coming in faster than he could answer them. I showed him a trick my senior resident had shown me, which was to keep a running list of the problems so that he wouldn't miss one, and could work the list the second there was a lull. I glanced over his shoulder as he scratched out the words: an infant running a fever in the emergency room who need to be admitted for a septic workup; a young girl on chemotherapy with intractable vomiting; a boy on the cardiac floor with a funny-looking rhythm on the monitor; and a mother with questions about her daughter in Room 376. As Kevin fell more and more behind I started responding to some of the pages, trying to take part of the load off him. With the workroom to ourselves he shook his head and let out a low whistle. "Living the dream," he said.

"Living the dream," I answered, smiling.

Part Three: Becoming

After the other ward teams had reported off their patients to us, we stopped by the wards and then rode the elevator down to the emergency room to examine the baby with the fever. The mother sat in the bed, mascara smudged under her eyes, her baby hugged close to her chest. She looked at us with apprehension. I nodded slightly to Kevin and he stepped up, placing his hand lightly on her shoulder, smiling confidently. "What a beautiful girl."

After Kevin took the history from the mother she stood in the hallway and I guided him as he performed a lumbar puncture. I hovered over him, pointing out the landmarks, double-checking the point at which he would insert the needle. I held my breath, but his hands were steady and sure. Clear fluid dripped from the needle into the tubes and after we were done, he ripped off his mask and gave me a high five. His grin seemed larger than anyone else's.

Later that night we sat in the workroom as I helped him through the paperwork, filling out the history and physical and getting orders in the computer. There was a knock on the door and Kevin's wife entered. Heidi was a neurology resident and she and Kevin were newly married. They fit perfectly, she as disarming as Kevin in her bright confidence, and I liked her immediately. We ate a quick dinner while fielding pages and discussing patients. For the first half of the night, we stayed together, working through each problem, but by two in the morning we were drowning. History and physical documentation, admission orders, and other issues were accumulating and we decided to split up.

About thirty minutes later, I was standing in the room of a bald four-year-old girl. *Ratatouille* played on the television overhead and she half-watched with listless eyes. Her mother lay on the daybed under the dark window. I tried to make a joke about the movie, but the girl had been vomiting half the night and seemed to look right through me. I had been feeling sorry for myself in my wrinkled white coat, with aching feet, already tired beyond comprehension with the night still young, but as I looked at her thin torso and the poisonous chemotherapy hanging from the IV pole I was awash in guilt. A moment later I was torn away by an urgent text page from Kevin: "Blood hitting ceiling, #344."

The windows blurred as I ran down the hall, heading for the east wing. I knew by the room number that the patient was on the surgical service—a group of patients we didn't cross-cover or get sign-out on. I burst through the door to find Kevin sitting on the bed with his hand in a small boy's mouth. Hanging from that mouth was the tail end of a piece of bright red gauze. The boy's mother sat on the other side of the bed, her arm around her son's shoulders; standing over her was the nurse.

"Had a tonsillectomy today!" Kevin blurted. "Just started bleeding out of the blue."

"Okay—can you page ENT?" I asked the nurse.

"Already did—he said to put pressure on it for a few minutes and then leave it be."

"He's not coming in?"

"No, he said to call him only if it didn't stop."

I looked at Kevin with his fingers all the way in the back of the boy's throat, the boy almost gagging. I looked at the fine spray of red on the ceiling. What were the chances that once we stopped holding pressure the bleeding wouldn't start back up? I looked around the room. "Okay, give me a second. I'm calling ENT."

I stepped out into the dimly lit hallway and called the resident at home. Instantly his voice unseated me, confident and condescending with a sort of Ivy League precision that made me want to appease him and make him believe I was on par with him. Instead, I stammered a few words: "We've got a kid with active bleeding, if . . ."

"Listen, it's just a bleeder from the scab getting scraped off. The kid probably dislodged the clot by eating or drinking—there's nothing to do. Just stop the bleeding and it will clot."

I had no argument, no credible experience. I hung up the phone, cursing under my breath. Kevin and I were alone on this one. I entered the room sheepishly and told them he wasn't coming in. Kevin looked at me, his eyes bright, a slight smile creasing the corner of his lips, and I knew immediately that it was in these types of situations that he was the most alive. There was nothing else to do. "Okay, Kevin, ease your fingers out. Let's see what happens."

The boy gagged softly as the gauze came out—if he vomited, the entire scab would come loose and the blood would come fast. I shone a light at the back of his throat and all I could see was beefy red, raw tissue, but no active bleeding. We waited five minutes to make sure the bleeding didn't resume, Kevin's pager continuing to beep until finally we left the room together.

"Nice job," I said. "You don't see that every day."

Kevin grinned his Cheshire grin. "Living the dream." As we walked down the hall, I thought about how when everyone else used that phrase it seemed laden with sarcasm and bitterness. Bitterness at a life on hold, at a decade of training, at a mountain of debt, at eighty-hour workweeks earning less than minimum wage. And yet with Kevin the expression rang true. The crazier things got, the happier he seemed. After being awake for thirty hours he wore the same grin, had the same gait down the hall, looked at me as if to say, "I can't believe we really get to do this."

Kevin and I worked together over that year and we developed a rhythm. He quickly became self-sufficient and our working relationship changed such that I became less of a supervising resident and more of a teammate. From the start, I had harbored my own insecurities. With his encyclopedic knowledge base, Kevin seemed to know more than I yet he always had a disarming smile and a certain humility. Most of all, he seemed to thrive under pressure and was always thankful and positive. At the same time, I could tell by the way he looked at me that he admired something in me, although I never knew what it could be.

After I completed my residency training, I stayed at the same hospital to do further training in neonatal medicine. Kevin became a senior resident under me during my time as a fellow and he truly shone in that role. He was always ready to teach and guide, always with that contagious grin. He gained a reputation for attracting the sickest patients—even on his outpatient months he ended up sending kids to the emergency room.

Late one afternoon he sauntered down the main hallway of the NICU, smiling and talkative. He was rotating through the pediatric ICU. I was slammed, but we talked briefly and he told me about some of the cases from the PICU. As always, he wore his characteristic smile and air of nonchalance. I couldn't help wishing I had the ability to seem so unaffected by the chaos around me.

"I'm thinking about applying for a PICU fellowship," he said.

"You sure you don't want to do neonatology?" I asked, knowing full well that his heart lay with pediatric ICU. "Just kidding—I can really see you doing PICU."

The respiratory therapist came up to us, handing me a slip of paper with an alarming blood gas. "Okay, I gotta go. Never a dull moment," I said, shaking my head as I walked away.

The next night I was on call overnight in the hospital. I sat at a bank of computers looking at an abdominal film when a young resident crumpled into a chair next to me, tears cascading off her cheeks, her lips quivering like a child's. Through her sobbing gasps I could make out that Kevin was dead; he had committed suicide. I looked at her and pitied her, for the terrible loss and seismic shift that I knew was underway. What I remember so vividly was my strength and clarity in that moment. I was unaffected, calm, and rational—I knew there had been a mistake. As the night wore on I talked with dazed residents and it angered me that they all said the same name, told the same story. In the NICU, the nurses offered me condolences as though I was grieving. I shrugged them off. I remained buoyed and resolute. Later that night, I closed the call room door behind me and the quiet settled in; I sat on the bed and tried to breathe.

Until that time suicide had always been something distant in my life. As a boy I was fascinated by a small motorcycle trophy my mother kept on her dresser. It had belonged to an uncle I never met. My family visited his grave once when I was a child, scraggy weeds crawling up the stone, the surrounding, scattered trees stripped and moss-covered. Much later, during training, I heard about a resident who had plunged from the rooftop several years before I started. The story haunted me, a testament to the toll that sleep deprivation, stress, and bearing witness to tragedy can take.

My memories of the days following Kevin's death appear as scraps. One night when my son had a fever, I drove out to the pharmacy for infant Tylenol. As I passed through my neighborhood, what had once felt charming and endearing felt empty and flat, as if there wasn't enough oxygen in the air, and I wondered how anything could ever be right in the world again. A few days later I was on a transport to get a sick baby from a small community hospital. We flew directly into the sunset and the orange light cast out over an ocean of green. I sat sequestered in my own world, cut off by the throb of the rotors and the tinted visor of my helmet. I looked at the perfect sunset with a brick in my throat as my eyes threatened to swim. I kept going over my last conversation with Kevin in the hallway, the guilt cresting over me—I should have known. *Why, why, why?* It was a mantra. Then, anger. *Why, damn it?* Then sorrow: I would have tried to help if I had known. And always, back to *why*. Was it the stress of the job? The senseless suffering that we were witness to as children and their families dealt with things that children should never have to confront—cancer, heart defects, immunodeficiency, and death? I wondered if I had ever really known him. How much of my experience of Kevin was of a shell that he had expertly built around himself?

The funeral took place in a chapel adjacent to gardens scattered with groves of loblolly pines, Japanese gardens of gentle streams and bamboo, ponds thick with white lilies and ridges of terraced flowers. Beyond the peace of the gardens rose the stone pinnacles of the university. I remember my first time visiting that garden. It was in the heady days at the start of training. My wife and I laid out a blanket on the grass for our five-month-old son and we sat together in the newness of the East Coast humidity, listening to the heavy drone of cicadas, enveloped in the green. Our son on his back, kicking his legs, the undergraduate campus and medical center just visible through the tops of the trees. Now I stood at these same gardens in a suit and tie, surrounded by black. The contrast between the young faces in black suits and dresses and the beautiful sunny day and lush garden made the whole thing seem improbable.

Even after all these years, thoughts of Kevin will blindside me with enough power to catch my breath. One spring morning, still fresh out of fellowship training, I pushed my daughter down the street on her tricycle. Above us the sky stretched out blue and cloudless, the trees green. Tulips dotted the neighbors' planters. I looked at my daughter's small body in the pink seat of the tricycle and inhaled the sticky sweet scent of fresh pollen. I thought of Kevin, of how he too could be walking down a street, done with the pressures of training, perhaps pushing his own child. I wondered where he would be, where he and Heidi would be living. It felt as though the night had passed and Kevin had never emerged.

Once, rummaging through a box in my closet, my fingers pressed into a pin that someone had made in remembrance of him. It has the sun shining through a cloud—the silver lining that he always saw in everything. With the cool metal of the pin in my hand, memories of that transport flight after Kevin died came back to me.

In my hurt and confusion, a song ran through my head. Over and over again, the refrain, "You make all things new" drowned out the helicopter blades and the crushing sense of loss. Now I see his face before me, grinning, feel the energy and excitement that always surrounded him and I know that I have more than a silver lining—I have a faith in a God who can restore broken babies and broken lives and make all things new.

Years later, I hold my daughter's hand as we walk across the atrium. It is a crisp day and the cold slips through my fleece like a sieve. Wooden tables and chairs flanked by boxes of flowers sit under the shadow of the nine-story hospital. We are alone.

The bench is just ahead, around the corner. I had forgotten the details—remembered it as a plain metal bench. In fact, the metal is purple-hued and in the center a green tree floats like the Tree of Life. Overhead the elm leaves flutter and my daughter asks, "Daddy why are we looking at this bench?"

I start to speak but my voice catches and falters.

"Are you going to cry?" she asks, her blue eyes searching and unsure.

"See the name on the bench?" I ask and her fingers trace the font as she sounds out the letters.

"He was a friend of mine."

"Did he die?"

"Yes sweetie, he did."

"How?"

"He got sick, baby."

"Oh, that would be like my friend Cora dying."

I can see figures moving through the glass and I think of this bench sitting here through the seasons, unnoticed by most, yet just standing in front of it threatens to drown me. I wonder who else visits; I think of his wife, his parents. I snap a picture of my daughter sitting there, so grown up since he last saw her, her rounded baby face now lean, her wavy blonde hair past her shoulders. Then I glance at the bench one last time, the purples and greens iridescent in the light, and push through the metal side gate into the throng of people at the hospital entrance, carried back into the present, my daughter's hand in mine.

Paige and Reese

The autumn day is crisp and windless, the light soft and smoky. We sit outside at a stone table, the hospital rising over our shoulders; I watch as people bustle along a glass-walled corridor. I feel no older now than when I first met Melissa six years ago and to me, she looks no different. Somehow it doesn't feel that long ago.

She sits with her volunteer bag beside her, one hour free until kindergarten pick up. I know pieces of the story. My life has intersected with hers at varying points, but I ask her to start at the beginning. She brushes a strand of hair behind her ear and when she speaks, I catch traces of Long Island.

It started almost seven years ago when, at twelve weeks, Scott and Melissa went in for the first ultrasound. The signs of pregnancy were few: a small, hard bulge in her lower abdomen, middling nausea, and sapping tiredness. She hadn't felt the baby move or kick. In a darkened room she lay on the exam table in a thin backless gown, the ties loose, the ultrasound gel cool and gelatinous as the probe slid across her skin. On the screen, a head lurched into view: a thin ribbon of skull, lakes of fluid lapping the brain cortex; the concavity of the ocular orbit running down into a ridge of nose; a thin neck and a heart fluttering like dragonfly wings; the potbelly distended; short, stubby legs with strands of bone; and, down the center of the back, the fine teeth of spine. They gazed at the screen and wondered. *Is that the head? Why is the stomach so big? Is everything okay?* Scott's chest tightened in anticipation as the pulsing heart came into view and a leg kicked and suddenly the idea of a baby morphed into something tangible. A minute later, the ultrasound technician smiled. "I'm hearing two heartbeats. Congratulations, you're having twins!"

Soon, grainy double forms came into view, floating in the black fluid. The technician scanned and re-scanned, measuring, punching in numbers, and squinting as she re-checked them. "Looks like you're having girls! I'll need some more pictures, but first I need you to get up and move around, do a circle around the room a few times, then touch your toes. We'll see if we can get them to move around a little so we can get some different views."

Again she scanned, pressing down, and rolling into the angles. She dragged lines across the screen, tapping the keys. Finally, she said, "Let me get the doctor."

In the quiet of the room, they tried to take it in.

"Twins," Scott said, grinning. "This is going to be a whole new ball game."

"Two," said Melissa. "Oh, wow! We need another name."

"What names do we have on the list?"

"Abby, Emma, Molly, Reese, and Paige."

"Okay, at least we have some to choose from."

"Oh, we need more stuff! We only have a single stroller. We're going to need a bunch of stuff—another crib, car seat, highchair. I don't know if Kamdyn's old clothes will be enough. Did we give some of them away already? How do you feed two babies?"

Scott shrugged and laughed.

The shuffling of papers, a crisp knock: Dr. Susan Janklow strode across the room, her handshake firm. There was a slight hesitation before she spoke, as if she were carrying a fine crystal vase over a stone floor. Melissa and Scott leaned forward, nervous and eager, already spinning with the news of twins, making plans and adjusting expectations, taking inventory of their resources—they had parents who lived in town, Scott could take a week or two off work, they could manage two babies, they could learn. Melissa thought of twins and of how the girls would always have a best friend, a confidante—they say twins are special soulmates, twins can talk in their own language, each twin knows what the other is thinking and feels what the other is feeling.

Dr. Janklow wanted to tell them gradually, carefully, but she couldn't dilute her words, and as she spoke, she had the sensation of pulling the air from their lungs. Baby B was small, two weeks behind on her growth already and much less developed than Baby A. There was a strong chance they could have twin-twin transfusion syndrome, a serious complication where abnormal blood vessels within the placenta couple the fetal circulations together, one twin drowning in blood flow while the other starves; there was a risk of brain damage, even death. Dr. Janklow said so many more words, but Melissa didn't hear them. She was silent, focused on a smudge in the carpet. Tears slipped over her cheekbones; she didn't notice Scott leaning over to ask if she was okay.

I imagine that night as they lay in bed, Melissa's head on Scott's shoulder, the moon shining through the blinds. It was late and quiet in the house. Melissa could tell from the regularity of Scott's breathing that he was still awake, staring at the ceiling.

"What are you thinking about?" she asked.

"Whether they're going to make it. I feel so powerless."

"Yeah, me too. I want to be strong and think positive but all I can think about is what she said—you know, brain damage and death."

"I know, I'm the same way. It's just such a shock—as if the surprise of twins wasn't enough, Baby B's so small. I guess all we can do is take it one day at a time and try to be calm—stress probably isn't good for them."

"You're right. I was wondering, should we name Baby B? I mean, since we don't know what's going to happen?"

"I'm not sure, but it seems strange not to name her."

"I agree, I want to name her—I think we should. I was thinking we could call her Reese. That way we can call her Reesie Piecey because she'll be so little."

"Yeah, that fits."

That night, worries followed Melissa into sleep, and she dreamed of small babies and doctor visits and bleeding. But when she woke in the morning, she whispered "Reese," and it made everything seem possible.

Melissa went in for ultrasounds three, sometimes four, times a week—forty-one ultrasounds in all. The ultrasounds became her life, her pregnancy so precarious they had to keep a constant watch on the growth of the babies and the pattern of flow in the umbilical cords. She couldn't stand to go alone. Each visit, while her almost three-year-old daughter Kamdyn colored pictures, ate goldfish crackers, or played on the preschool playground, Melissa sat in the passenger seat, the lap belt snug under the fold of her abdomen, thinking of growth and wondering how far the pregnancy would go. Over and over, she heard Dr. Janklow's echoing words, "You know, you might come in one day and hear only one heartbeat—or none." During one visit, the doctor offered termination; Melissa shook her head.

Perhaps she glanced at the faces in the cars beside her as they traveled to grocery stores or coffee dates or the dry cleaners, her mind heavy with apprehension and foreboding. Hands gripping her purse, jaw muscles tight, arriving at the hospital without knowing how she got there. Most days, she saw families leaving with their newborns, the car under the shade of the overhang, the baby carefully loaded into the car seat, and she remembered taking Kamdyn home, almost three years to the day. She longed for the simplicity and newness of those days. She longed for the first years of marriage when she and Scott came home from work and cooked together, trying out new recipes, and then ate on the little balcony of their apartment while the neighbor's country music played below. It wasn't jealousy she felt when she saw families leaving the hospital, but a deep river of longing and the sensation of being older and somehow separate.

Soon Melissa knew everyone in the maternal-fetal center, especially Mary, her ultrasonographer. Each visit she watched as Mary brought the images onto the screen, grays and blacks and whites flashing into view, grainy and amorphous, like fog, like the way clouds shift and stream past a plane window. To Melissa, Mary's face was an auspice: she followed each expression, each click as the ultrasonographer measured, wondering what the verdict would be. Mary chatted as she worked, telling Melissa about her daughter's softball game in Charleston, the amount of homework they were giving in seventh grade, how the middle-schoolers were vaping in the bathrooms. For brief moments, the chatting put Melissa at ease and drew her attention from the screen.

"Have you picked names yet?"

"Yes, we knew the day of the first scan that we would name Baby B Reese, but we couldn't decide for Baby A, so we had a family vote. Paige won out."

"Oh, how cute! Those are great names—they go together."

Each scan, Paige grew steadily, tracking along the 55th percentile. She moved and kicked; the blood flow in her umbilical cord rose and fell into peaks and valleys, jets of red and blue, nutrients and oxygen coursing through to her growing body. Each scan, Reese was so small she couldn't be plotted on the growth chart, but she spun and wriggled. Her cord hung slightly off to the side of the placenta and, within its thin walls the blood flowed intermittently, not in jets but as attenuated sighs.

The ultrasound appointments continued until twenty-six weeks when the diastolic flow in Reese's umbilical cord slowed to a dribble and Dr.

Janklow admitted Melissa to the hospital for steroid shots, bed rest, and constant monitoring. Melissa pauses as she gets to this part of our shared history. I wonder how her impressions and memory will correlate with mine. She smiles.

"Our nurse told us you were the new guy. You had just finished training. We felt bad for you."

This is what I remember: I took the stairs down to the antenatal floor and hesitated outside Room 172. I knew the way the door would open, the upside-down latch cool to my fingers and the wood stuck to the paint of the frame, causing me to nudge with my shoulder until it gave way. The hand sanitizer dispenser would ratchet down, squeezing the chemical foam into my hand outstretched in supplication. The mother would be in bed, perhaps with a phone pressed to her ear and a plate of food on a plastic tray in front of her. I wondered if the knock at the door would startle her. I suspected she already knew, low and deep, that we could save one of her babies but not the other.

A blue-and-white gown and a blond ponytail. A canvas tote by the window, and the muffled double beats of the babies' hearts on the monitor. Tracks of paper spilled from the machine. Scott rose to shake my hand and I rolled a stool towards the bedside.

"So, I bet you weren't expecting to end up here today!"

"No, I was in for my routine scan and then they admitted me straight from clinic."

"I know it's a surprise. Do you live close? Do you have other kids?"

"Yes, we're pretty close, just fifteen minutes away. We have Kamdyn— she's almost three."

"You have your hands full! Do you have names picked out?"

"Yes, Paige for A and Reese for B."

I started with the easy part, giving them the facts: the location of the NICU, visiting hours, and who to expect at delivery. But soon my words wound through the lexicon of critical care: breathing tubes, central lines, risk of intraventricular hemorrhage, chronic lung disease, and necrotizing enterocolitis. Melissa seemed to recede into herself as I went over the potential complications. I inched closer to the truth, backing away at the last minute. I'm sure they could see it; I just needed a way to start.

"As you know, Reese is really small. Unfortunately, she's too small right now for our equipment—I don't think the breathing tube would fit."

Melissa smiled bravely, tears catching the light while Scott dragged his chair closer to hold her hand.

"Have you ever had a baby this small survive?" Melissa asked.

I thought of twins born during my training, both at just over 300 grams. I remembered the way their skin sloughed off after the second day and they got septic. We ramped up the blood pressure drips, gave steroids and antibiotics, until bleeding swelled their brains and bacteria overwhelmed their bloodstreams. They clung to life for over a week and a half before their hearts stopped beating.

"No, unfortunately not at this weight."

"What will happen to her? What if she tries to breathe?" asked Melissa.

"We'll place her on your chest so you can hold her. If it looks as though she's struggling, we can give her some morphine to make her more comfortable."

I left the room heavyhearted—it didn't seem enough just to care or wish it were different. It felt like a betrayal to tell them that we could do nothing and then fall right back into the patterns of my daily life; to drive home, eat dinner, wash dishes, and read bedtime stories to my children. At the periphery of my mind, just over the flimsily constructed fence, lapped feelings of impotence, failure, and guilt. But I knew well enough how the line between compassion and futility blurs.

Four days into the hospital admission Kamdyn turned three, and as Melissa lay in bed, Scott managed the Little Gym party. Melissa worried about the details—would Scott remember to pick up the cake, would he take enough pictures, and could he get Kamdyn's hair done right? But he managed to pull it off and the children ran barefoot over the mats, bounced off the springboards and leapt into the foam ball pit. The cake had pink frosting. There were princess goodie bags for each child to take home. After the party Kamdyn came to the hospital in a billowing, lacy dress, long purple gloves, and a plastic sparkly tiara. She was tall in her plastic high heels, her calves thin and poised. She crawled in next to Melissa and snuggled under her arm. They opened cards and presents together, the wrapping paper littering the bed, and Scott snapped pictures. Later, they had a picnic dinner in the room before Scott drove Kamdyn home for a bath and bedtime.

As Melissa tells me this part of the story, I think of my own daughters playing dress-up, the click of plastic heels on the wooden floor, and of holding them close, the glitter falling off the tinseled dresses onto my shirt, their little bodies regal and earnest and soft all at once. Of how, when I squeeze them, they squirm and tell me that hugging them is not a part of the game. I think then that I will always hold them close even when they are grown. And as I look at Melissa, I think of the night I first met her, in her fifth year of marriage, college not such a distant memory, and of how we all at some point cross the shadow line from the naïveté of youth.

Pictures of a younger me belie the years that slip by, the changes accumulating gradually. I wish my children could have seen me before these changes, when I was in college or in my early twenties. The man I want them to see is captured in a picture from my grandparents' back garden in New Zealand. In the picture I stand tanned, thick-haired, and broad-shouldered. My eyes are sure and strong, unflinching with optimism. That was before the days and nights when uncertainty leaked through the slats and pieces of heartache thrummed against the casings. The man I see in pictures now has creases of vulnerability, not only for himself but for others.

After a week of monitoring, Reese's blood flow looked slightly better and they let Melissa go home. At first, she was afraid to slip from the monitor, to leave the reassuring smiles of the nurses and a hospital room where a doctor was never more than fifty yards away. She wondered if she could break bed rest to shower. I picture her on the drive home, gazing out the window as the trees skidded by, sunlight flickering across her face. When they pulled up to the house it was familiar and warm and her time in the hospital seemed somehow distorted. On Monday, Scott went to work and Kamdyn to school and the house was still. Sunlight streamed through the blinds in the morning, casting shadows; a lawnmower droned outside, and pine branches clicked as they flexed in the breeze.

Seven weeks of bed rest. Seven weeks of directing traffic from the bed or couch, unable to take Kamdyn to preschool, grocery shop, make dinner, or walk the neighborhood. Midway through the seven weeks, during an ultrasound visit, it looked as though the flow in Reese's umbilical vessels had reversed. Instead of flowing through the umbilical cord into the placenta as it should, each time her heart squeezed, the abnormally high pressure in the placenta sent the blood backwards, like the tide sucking back into the sea. She was in danger of acid buildup and death.

Again, Melissa found herself in a hospital bed, her mother-in-law sitting next to her. Scott drove fast to the hospital, parked out front, pushed the elevator button five times, and ran down the hallway. He arrived breathless, his face red, a shoelace untied. It turned out to be a false alarm. When they re-scanned her before C-section surgery, the flow in the umbilical cord looked better. They said she could go home but fear lapped against her and she chose to return to her hospital room where she ate soggy, salted hospital food and stared out at the air-conditioning units on the gravel roof.

She went home the next morning and time resumed its previous form—the hollowed-out days of waiting, moments that hinged on the door flying open as Kamdyn burst into the mudroom, dropped her backpack, and raced over to the couch, then later the bustle of her mother in the kitchen and the sound of Scott slipping his keys on the hook by the door.

Dr. Janklow scheduled the C-section for 34 weeks, telling her, "Reese will grow better out of the womb and the chance of survival is much better than before."

By 34 weeks, Paige weighed 5.6 pounds and Reese was just big enough for tubes and lines. Melissa remembers the delivery as a blur of images and impressions: staring up at the white tiles of the OR ceiling; the sharp pain of the IV needle; and the familiar, reassuring voice of her obstetrician. Paige came out first and she cried right away. Dr. Janklow held her up over the drape so Melissa could see her. Drops of blood and amniotic fluid dripped down on Melissa and she smiled up at Paige's red face and pouting lip. Melissa didn't hear Reese cry, but the neonatologist came over after a few minutes and said the breathing tube went in without any problems. Scott took a picture of Reese, thin-boned and tiny on the warmer, then carried Paige in his arms as he walked beside the team wheeling Reese to the NICU.

That afternoon, Melissa shimmied out of bed and into a wheelchair and Scott wheeled her down to the NICU. From the first day, she could hold Paige. Her body was warm against Melissa's chest and her hair smelled softly of baby shampoo; she could hear the rhythmic sigh of the CPAP machine inhaling and exhaling. She opened the porthole of the incubator and slipped a finger into her other daughter's palm. Five pieces of plastic entered Reese's body: an endotracheal tube, a nasogastric tube, a central arterial line, a central venous line, and a scalp IV.

On day three, Dr. Janklow wrote the discharge order and the nurse helped Melissa down to the lobby. "That was one of the hardest days," she tells me. "How are you supposed to leave your babies alone in the hospital?"

I shake my head, "Honestly, I don't know."

Her C-section scar continued to close in on itself, that part of her past already fading. She couldn't drive for two weeks and every day Scott drove her to the hospital, where she sat in a recliner between the two incubators and watched the nurses measure yellow breast milk into feeding syringes, string IV fluids, and tap on the computer keyboards. Paige moved through the steps methodically, as if checking off boxes. She weaned off CPAP, tolerated tube feedings, came off IV fluids, and then, a week later, started taking her feeds by mouth. When she was seventeen days old, they carried her down to the lobby. The welcome desk was empty and the sun coming through the glass sliding doors was bright. Scott pulled the minivan up to the curb, clipped the car seat into the base, and they headed for home. Everything felt familiar. Paige drank her bottles, dozed in Melissa's arms, and smiled in her sleep.

With Reese, everything was new and different: ventilators, blood gases, electrolytes, parenteral fluids, nasogastric feedings, ampicillin, gentamicin, head ultrasounds, infections, and a cleft palate. I think that every time the phone rang, fear must have surged up from Melissa's stomach, spreading up to her throat, and when she answered her vocal cords were tight, her voice high and edgy.

Melissa's description matches my memory. Time passed and Reese slowly grew. In the early days there were some gains—she came off the ventilator, tolerated tube feedings, and weaned off IV fluids and medications. After a month she was ready to attempt feeding from a bottle. The first time, she pushed out her tongue, scrunched up her face; milk dribbled from the corner of her mouth. As time went by, she improved little from her first attempts; days crawled into weeks, and what little gains she made one day she lost the next. Each time she fed, she would suck for a few minutes then pinch her lips, throw her head to the side, and refuse to take more. Sometimes when she fed, she sputtered, her heart rate dropped, and they had to stop and reposition her. The speech therapist worried about aspiration. In the radiology suite they fed her milk laced with barium and watched as minute amounts of the mixture slipped past her vocal cords. They added ground oatmeal and tried again until the thickness was right and the sludgy concoction moved from her throat to her esophagus to her stomach. But even with the new mixture, her feeding volumes remained low. After all the barriers that had loomed like mountain peaks before them and were now in the distance, it came down to one thing: feeding. No matter how much they tried to coax her, to whisper encouragement and cheer her on, she shut down after several minutes as if someone had flipped a switch and turned off the light.

That part of the hospitalization was marked by the slow passage of time, and with an absence of any perceivable forward momentum, it seemed as if there was no end in sight. After 67 days my colleague called a family meeting. They sat in the conference room, around the oversized table, the walls a yellowed white and just through the window, the sun shining on the outside world. The social worker started talking, then the doctor took over, laying out a new plan. "Reese isn't really making any progress on her feeding. At this rate she won't be ready to go home for a long time—six months, maybe more. She needs a more permanent way of getting her feeds."

She told them about the possibility of placing a feeding tube that Reese could go home with, a G-tube. The tube would be placed by a pediatric surgeon and track from inside Reese's stomach to outside. Scott and Melissa would be able to hang a feeding pouch, attach the tubing to the outside button, and let gravity draw the milk into her stomach. Once Reese no longer needed the G-tube, it could be removed. She would end up with a little scar over her stomach. The doctor explained that the surgery would have to be done at another hospital because they didn't have a pediatric surgeon there. "The good thing is that you'll be able to take her home after several days."

They looked at each other—a new hospital, anesthesia, surgery.

Scott said to Melissa, "It would get her home."

Melissa thought of the empty crib and nodded.

Now, as Melissa tells me about their time in the NICU, I realize that details have sifted from her memory—the time Reese spent in the hospital is more of a feeling or sensation than the objective measure of discrete moments. Melissa can't remember how many days Reese stayed on the ventilator or what the doctors first told her about the cleft palate or possible bloodstream infection. What she remembers is an IV burrowed into Reese's scalp, the tubing tracking from the infusion pump, threading through a port of the incubator, tunneling through her daughter's fine sandy hair, through her thin, pink skin. Melissa knew it stopped just under the surface of the skin, but it looked as though it went deeper, and the thought made her shudder. She also remembers a day, just as she was leaving the bedside, when Reese stopped breathing, her heart rate fell, and she turned blue. Her nurse picked her up and slapped her back, saying, "Reese, Reese, come on, get with the program, honey." Tears slid down Melissa's face, and Reese breathed.

I wonder what another parent in the room might have thought as they sat at their baby's bedside and saw the event unfold. I wonder what it's like to see the pain in another parent's eyes and to worry something like that could happen to your baby. Do families notice when we wheel new babies down the hall, our fast steps cushioned in OR booties? When we hurriedly assemble in an adjacent room, voices raised, slamming open the drawers of metal carts or trundling the X-ray machine down the hall? If Melissa saw those things, they have since trickled from her memory. The only lasting impressions now are those of walking to the pumping room and then back to the bedside; of the equipment surrounding Reese; of the calming support of the nurses and the ever-present sensation of a heavy weight enveloping her body.

Three years after she left the hospital, I ran into Melissa at the Little Gym after my daughter's class. I smiled as Reese marched by me to a table of crayons, grabbed a coloring book, and sat intently coloring a princess picture, her legs dangling from the chair. Paige sat next to her, still twice her size. Melissa and I stood by the table and she filled me in on the last few years.

"Reese got the G-tube and came home pretty quickly after that—just a few days, really. At first, she took some of her feedings by mouth, but when she was ten months old she had to have cleft palate surgery. She totally shut down after that. Her feeding therapists tried everything—chin support, reflux medicines, thickened feeds."

Despair mounted as months accumulated into years and still Reese refused to eat. "She's just so stubborn. When she doesn't want to eat, she tightens her teeth and says, 'Hook me up.'"

They couldn't help but wonder if she would ever eat. Melissa heard about a six-week feeding program run by a university three hours away. It would mean time apart from Scott, Kamdyn, and Paige, but it just might work. Just after Reese's second birthday, Melissa packed up the car, loaded her in, and drove east. Miraculously, a group of young psychology students helped Reese start eating again.

The other concern was her small size. Despite a high-calorie diet, her growth lagged. They tried to increase calories with protein shakes, but she hated every flavor and getting her to drink was like going into battle. They tried every high-calorie food they could think of: ice cream, avocados, cheese, yogurt. Melissa laughed, "She seems to have a goal to burn as many calories a day as possible. She runs everywhere, climbs constantly—we keep having to stop ourselves from telling her, 'Don't do that honey, you'll burn calories.' And we still don't know why she's so tiny. All the genetic tests were negative. We tried growth hormone shots, but it didn't work and she was so miserable. Finally, Scott said 'Enough—she's not an experiment!' We just decided to let her be."

As we stood talking, I felt an irrational sense of responsibility, as though I should have known this would happen and, more importantly, should have prevented it. Perhaps I felt it all the more sharply because while we talked, my daughter Avery sat next to Reese and as I watched them color I thought of all the uncertainty and worry that Scott and Melissa had to face that I didn't. And even though I was no longer her doctor it seemed that I should know the answers and how to fix the problem.

Another three years have gone by and now, sitting with Melissa at the stone table outside the hospital, she tells me that Paige and Reese started kindergarten. I picture them posing for a first-day-of-school picture, standing on the driveway in front of a boxwood, the summer sun already cresting the trees. Paige in a blue and white dress, her hair pulled back into a ponytail, and an arm draped around Reese's shoulder. Reese weighs almost twenty-three pounds, half the size of her sister.

"What are their personalities like? Are they similar?" I ask Melissa.

"Even though they're twins, they're so different! Paige takes her time and loves to be fancy. She's so motherly—sometimes when I'm in the other room I hear them playing and have to tell her, 'Paige, same age.' She treats Reese like she's her little sister."

I laugh. "My girls are the same way."

"Reese can be pretty stubborn. She's fiercely independent. If someone says something about her size, she tells them, 'I'm not small.'"

"Does she still have the G-tube?"

"Yes—we've only used it a couple of times this past summer. We keep thinking we should have it taken out but it's our safety net."

I think of Reese getting her tube feeds at home, curled up on the couch, tucked under a pink blanket; the TV playing low, light flickering across the room and her pump ticking, squeezing 300 mL of milky white fluid in over 1.5 hours. After the feed they carry her into the bedroom, trying not to wake Paige.

I glance at my watch. I have a meeting and it's time for Melissa to head to the school pick up line. As I walk down the hallway, I am struck by how easy things would have been, the first night I met Scott and Melissa, if I had known then what I know now. If I could have stepped outside of time and walked along the glass corridor and looked out to see myself at the table with Melissa in the fall sunlight. If I could have seen that picture from the first day of kindergarten. I could have breathed a sigh of relief and reassured Scott and Melissa that everything would be okay. Now six years later, Melissa tells me, "We've come a long way—we are a normal family now."

The weather turns, there is frost on the grass in the mornings, and the leaves have all but blown from the trees. I knock on another hospital door. Maysha Connally is carrying twins and, like Melissa's girls, one is growing well while the other is severely growth-restricted. Maysha sits in bed. Her nails click the glass of her phone as she looks up at me through long black lashes; I know her.

"You took care of Jayla three years ago when she was in the NICU," she tells me.

"Yes, that's right—I knew I recognized you."

"She's so big now, she's doing great. Want to see a video of her?"

She swipes her fingers across the screen until she finds a clip and holds it out for me. I see a toddler with black curly hair and a plastic tube in her throat careening across the living room, the images blurring with the speed.

"You probably remember, she went home with a trach—she just goes on the vent overnight."

I remember Jayla, small and fragile, and none of my memories correlate with the girl in the video.

Now Maysha is back and in her womb, one baby absorbs nutrients and fattens while the other starves, the blood flow from the umbilical cord sluggish and hesitant. Any day, the inadequacy of that blood flow could snuff out the baby girl's life, and the immune reaction to her death would place her brother in jeopardy. Any day the circular plastic monitor, held in place with stretched gauze, could threaten impending collapse and they would rush Maysha down the halls to the C-section suite.

Sitting next to her, with the afternoon sun coming through the window and falling on my face, the hum of the intermittent pneumatic compression device squeezing her calves, I harbor two selves. One the eternal optimist who remembers Paige and Reese, explaining dire reality to Melissa and Scott, telling them we couldn't save Reese—and then how Reese made it, staying in the womb until she was big enough, and is now in kindergarten. I have countless other stories, some more harrowing but with great outcomes. I have seen these babies at reunions, at the grocery store, and at soccer games. Then there is the other self, the one that has seen what happens when the pregnancy doesn't go as planned, wished, or prayed. And upon this self lies the heavy burden of warning. We don't know why one pregnancy goes on, uninterrupted, while another comes crashing to a halt. Almost every mother asks, "What did I do?" I tell them the same thing: "You did nothing wrong. There was nothing you could do to stop this."

I think back to when I first met Scott and Melissa, of my guilt and inability to help, of the time Reese spent in the NICU, of the next six years of her life and of what transpired. I think of the moments when the future was uncertain, foggy, and the terrain seemed to shift and buckle. I couldn't make any promises. The first night we met, I left Reese's parents scared and anxious like a couple looking at an oncoming hurricane. Now I have a vantage point and the vista is clear. And yet again, I am in the same place, sitting in a room with a mother, the future entirely uncertain. The fetal monitor beeps and the light from her phone reflects off her glasses. Seconds to minutes, minutes to hours, hours to days, the weight of the past pressing into the future, and all we can see is the wake in the distance and the possibilities ahead.

All Things New

We travel a one-lane road, folding up over the curve of a hill. We pass farms of mowed grass, clumps yellowing in the sun, scatterings of pink blossomed trees. A wooden barn flanks a line of white fence, a painted American flag fading on the side, and further on, a dock juts over the algae-lined edge of a pond. Above it all, the spring sun is crisp and vivid.

My wife sits beside me, and we are quiet. Her face is turned toward the window, and I wonder if she is crying. It is a strange time. A surreal time. Even now, as I guide the car down the road, an invisible plague is moving across the land; each day the death count rises and what once seemed far away is now in our midst. Yesterday, we heard about a man from church, a husband and father, who was admitted to the ICU at the hospital where I work. Today we found out he is dead. It happened just after lunchtime. His quarantined wife, now a widow, pressed her hand against the glass as her friend prayed from the other side. The spring of 2020 is a time like no other in our lives.

Driving in silence, under the weight of someone else's sorrow, I think of a story I have clung to all these years, a story that has sustained me through times of grief.

People sometimes ask me how I cope with the heartbreaking realities of working in the ICU. In those moments I think of Sam: of how his family taught me about redemption; of how his story changed the way I see the world. And of how his is a story for us all.

A decade ago, one early summer evening, I made my way down the polished hallway, knocked softly on the wooden door, and clicked the metal lever up.

The door swung inwards and the room smelled of fried chicken and potatoes. The window let in the softening light; outside, an oak gathered the last of the languid heat, and inside, the muffled cry of a woman in labor seeped through the walls. Clara Thomas—freckled, with strawberry-blonde hair, clear bluish-gray eyes, and long, thin arms—sat propped up in a hospital bed. In every way she fit her persona as a preschool teacher. On the daybed under the window, flanked by two small boys, sat her husband, Mark. He rose to greet me, tanned in a T-shirt, frayed jeans, and flip-flops. Clara mustered a weak smile, her face flushed and clammy, discreet white pearl earrings catching the fluorescent light. The boys colored in small workbooks, occasionally glancing up at me.

The atmosphere was incongruent with the circumstances. Clara was in her twenty-seventh week of pregnancy, but her abdomen threatened to expel the baby. Droplets of clear medicine were infused into her bloodstream to stave off the contractions; no one knew when she would deliver. I had only about ten minutes to meet the family and explain prematurity, its complications, the chances of survival, and what to expect in the delivery room and during a NICU hospitalization. The phone on my hip continued to ring—the NICU was filled to capacity and I had a running list of issues that grew each minute.

There were no extra chairs and I leaned hard against the wall, taking as much weight off my feet as possible. While I talked, sweat muddied Clara's foundation and Mark looked up at her from the coloring book. In our hospital, we often cared for babies who were delivered as early as 23 weeks; on average, 75 percent of those babies died. At 27 weeks, Mark and Clara's baby had a chance of survival in the high 80s, which from my frame of reference was pretty good, though if that were my son I don't know if I could breathe.

The rest of the evening was consumed by managing the usual host of issues in the NICU: adjusting ventilators, low blood pressure, low urinary output, apnea, and heart rate dips. Just before eleven, I hauled myself through the cafeteria and emerged with a plastic tray of sushi, salt-and-vinegar potato chips, and a Styrofoam cup of tepid coffee. I ate cross-legged on the call room bed, relishing the quiet and the taste of food. Monet prints were attached to the walls, eye laser equipment occupied one corner, and journals littered the desk. I was thirty years old and this was my life.

By two in the morning I slid between the thin, bleached sheets, fully clothed, with my socks and shoes set out at the side of the bed, and dropped off the cliff into a dreamless sleep. An hour later the phone shrieked into the blackness—Clara Thomas was in labor.

Her son, Sam, was tiny and blue and fatless. A bald, oversized head, skinny ribs, and thin splayed limbs. His abdomen sunken, his skin translucent, and his chest still. We squeezed air into his lungs and when I listened with a stethoscope, all I could hear was the coarse crackling of wet sticky lungs—no heartbeat. His father stood five feet behind my left shoulder and the nurse started chest compressions while I slipped a breathing tube through the vocal cords. While the respiratory therapist squeezed air and oxygen through the tube, I listened again and the heartbeat came to me like a distant train, so faint at first as to be just the murmur of the thing to come, then more surely. Next, we dripped milky white surfactant into his lungs, watching the heart rate on the monitor as it stalled, then took hold again. Behind me, the useless placenta slipped into a blue bowl. Beads of sweat dotted my hairline. Mark Thomas shifted uneasily.

Across the room, in the dimness, I could see Clara: face drained of blood; eyes fixed on her baby, loving and gentle.

I wheeled the transport incubator, erratically veering off course from time to time with the rubber wheels spinning sideways like a shopping cart, while the respiratory therapist faithfully squeezed air into Sam's lungs and his father followed in our wake. Sam's body was cocooned in a clear plastic bag to keep the heat in, his blue-gray wrinkled face emerging from under the plastic, a miniature blue-striped beanie meeting his downy eyebrows. I could see the fragments of blue tributary veins threading under his eyelids. A dusting of thin blond hair creased the ridge of his cheeks. I made small talk as we walked, hoping to build rapport as Mark told me their story.

Mark and Clara dreamed of a baby and the years went by, infertility treatments and shards of dreams. As he talked, I found myself flashing back to when my wife and I tried for a baby—the way time stretched out, each month's negative test morphing into what seemed like a year. For us it was only a short time, yet for them it was years. I could picture them driving silently together to the infertility clinic, their guilt and frustration almost suffocating. I could see Mark's hand reaching for Clara's taut knee with something pressing into his chest before Clara changed into a backless gown and the needle slid into her.

After several years of doctor's visits they adopted Abai, a two-year-old boy from Ethiopia. Then two years later in China, Hui toddled over to them and they scooped him up and carried him out of the orphanage. Shortly after their plane touched down from Beijing, cells so small as to be invisible buried into the boggy tissue of Clara's uterus and this time, miraculously, took hold.

Mark spoke with an easiness, the heartache borne completely without resentment—everything exactly the way it was supposed to be, everything in its right place, everything blessed. And as we traveled the pale, lonely halls he carried that certainty with him into this night as well.

Several hours later, Clara sat in a wheelchair and Mark wheeled her down the stretches of hallways and through the partially occupied waiting room. They washed hands at a large porcelain sink and moved down the hallway looking for Pod 5, their faces taut with sickening anticipation in the dimness and quietness.

Mark and Clara rounded the corner into the pod, and I watched them anxiously scan the room for their baby until their gaze rested on me standing over Sam's incubator. Machines blinked all around, tubes and wires interlaced and muddled; they stood frozen, with the strangeness cresting over them. Then, as if sleepwalking, Mark pushed the wheelchair into the room, the six incubators jutting out from the wall like piers, the nurses sliding noiselessly, the miniature flashes of drip rates on the pumps. Around us the flicker of the fluorescent lights, the gentle shifting of a sleeping baby and the sudden piercing of an alarm, the sloppy gurgling of water in ventilator tubing.

Clara seemed to see none of it. When she first saw Sam, it was as if the world disconnected, everything but Sam faded and immaterial. The light glared off the plastic of the incubator and warm humid air fogged the inside. Vapor intermittently misted the bore of the breathing tube. Sam did not move except for the even rise and fall of his small barrel chest.

My eyes felt like sandpaper, my mouth dry and sour. Just two more hours until the day would begin and reinforcements would arrive. The blood pressure numbers flashed red, a slow beeping emerging from the machine. I tried a weak smile, meant to be reassuring—my eyes met the nurse's, worry visible in the fine creases around her eyes. Milliliters of clear medication traveled the hollow of the catheter before dissolving in the crush of his bloodstream. A heart the size of a walnut, fed by hair-thin vessels, innervated by a spider's web of nerve fibers. More medicine: blood pressors, antibiotics, fluids. The pressure in his vessels transiently rose only to bank down again.

Outside the windowless intensive care unit dawn emerged, pink rimming the clouds, a lazy humidity enveloping the world. I sat in a chair by the bedside, grew impatient, and blundered around the room, heavy and helpless. At six in the morning the cafeteria unfurled the metal barricades. I sat at a table under the corrugated glass skylight, feeling night and day merge into one. The coffee was warm and familiar. I thought of my own family waking into the new day and wondered what this day would bring for Sam. My dazed reverie was broken by my pager—his blood pressure was tracking down.

We sat in a triangle. Clara looked exhausted to the point of inexpression. I said the words about the ventilator and blood pressure and antibiotics and bloodstream infection. To my own ears, they sounded technical and flat. Mark's eyes were raw and tender, focused on Clara's face. Mark grasped her hand, but she did not close her fingers over his. I pictured myself and Danielle in these chairs; I wanted to somehow reach across the invisible line and show them how deeply I cared.

I once heard of a cardiothoracic surgeon who was brilliant, and often drunk, who was checking on a baby after surgery. The baby wasn't doing well, so the surgeon ripped off the monitors, scooped the baby up and ran straight to the operating room. I wanted to be that surgeon—to scoop up the baby and run with my feet slapping the ground, the hospital blurring, the future yielding to me.

But instead, I sat. I told them that we were doing everything possible for their son, and then I had no other words. Behind me, Sam's nurse tapped on the keyboard until my lack of words grew uncomfortable and I excused myself. Retreating, I glanced back at Clara and in that moment, she looked old-fashioned and tragic and elegant.

I returned to the room about an hour later and the whole family was gathered around the incubator. Mark was holding his now-middle son, Hui, up and over the plastic, while his other son, Abai, was tall enough to peer in, at eye level with his new brother. Clara stood in hospital-issue socks, the lone female in the family, one hand resting softly on the face of the incubator. That sense of warmth I had felt in their hospital room now occupied the space around them. I tried to identify its elements but knew only that I sensed a lightness and comfort. Mark kissed the nape of Hui's neck, Abai breathed words to Sam, and Clara absentmindedly stroked Abai's hair.

I was slow to accept it—as if my unacceptance could make it not so. Sam was dying. All the numbers told me so and I hated them. It seemed impossible, with all the technology, all the research and journal articles, and all the medical expertise that existed within the hospital, that we would lose Sam that morning.

Nurses, pharmacists, doctors, parents bustled through the room. Babies cried in sudden fits of hunger and then sipped milk contentedly; alarms rang and were silenced. The day progressed, oblivious, as a family's dream slipped away.

Then the monitors never stopped flashing and Sam looked blue and spent. Mark sat on a chair and pulled a boy onto each knee. Clara sat beside him. In the busyness of the room, his arms enveloped the boys and he explained that Sam was too sick to come home to their house—instead, he would go straight to heaven. And it was in heaven that they would all be reunited. Sam would love heaven and be waiting for them.

While I stood to the side, searching in vain for another medicine, another option, Mark prayed, his voice reaching up to pull heaven down into the room. He was so sure of where Sam was going. He knew that it was a good place and that he would see Sam again. I thought of my own son playing with trains at his small train table, of shoes on damp autumn leaves and toothy grins, and then blinked and turned my face away.

Not long afterwards I sat at a long table of a restaurant, nestled in the mellow hills of California, surrounded by my extended family. Out in the meadow horses grazed in the golden pre-sunset light, the leaves in the oaks rippled in the breeze; the manicured grass in front of the restaurant was impossibly green.

My son sat in his high chair, contorting his mouth into garbled nonsense words, the floor around him strewn with pieces of pasta and speckled with Parmesan cheese. He finished his dinner early and strained against the chair's straps. My wife took him outside to the grass and I watched them through the window, his feet pumping across the lawn, her dress flowing back. Tears streamed without warning down my cheeks. I waded to the bathroom and splashed water on my face. I stood dripping and confused, my eyelids red and thick, smudges of gray under my eyes.

It seemed complicated that evening in the restaurant, with family all around and out the window soft greens and yellows, with a softening coolness drafting in the door when it was opened—everyone together, faces from my life, those who knew me before I ever watched a baby die. And me, comforted by their presence, yet isolated by my experiences. I had carried the memories with me on the flight to California, on the drive up the coast and along a ribbon of road winding through the golden hills—they clung to me, I could feel them against my skin. With the cool slip of my dinner jacket's sleeve against my wrist and the light dipping over the corral, I swam under a disquieting strangeness. In my chest I carried a heaviness, layer upon layer of memories: one day, Mark prayed with a boy on each knee as his son slipped away; the next, I was surrounded by family and beauty. Though I had left behind the shrill sound of bedside alarms, the acrid smell of disinfectant drying on the floor, and the windowless artificial light, two disparate worlds coalesced and I couldn't hold them at the same time without cracking; each overwhelmed the other. I had the sensation of coming home to find everything changed, yet the only thing changed was me.

I pushed out the heavy double doors and stood watching my wife and son, and the complexity and heaviness drained away.

I had a glimpse of heaven; of standing in the presence of God; of parents watching their children run with restored bodies, when all becomes new.

Epilogue

I sit with a mother as her baby's body shuts down, every organ failing one by one. A runnel of tears makes a line down her cheeks; the beads fall heavy on her thin hospital gown. "Why did this happen to me? I'm a good person, I try to do everything right. What did I do wrong? What is God trying to teach me?"

It's a question I've heard again and again, phrased a hundred different ways. And it's the same question that haunted me as I sat in church years ago, as the voices around me sang of God's goodness, the words glancing off my unconvinced heart.

As I sit by her bed, I want to share a litany of ideas that have transformed me over the years: God did not do this to you; you didn't do anything wrong. To tell her God is entirely good and loving and all-powerful, yet we live in a world punctured by immense pain and brokenness and darkness. That every life has meaning, no matter how short the time is. Tension and mystery—they are ours to embrace.

But in that moment she doesn't need my words; she needs my hand in hers. For we, despite our fragility and brokenness, are called to be obedient to the ageless call to love our neighbor, the person right in front of us. There will be a time later to tell her God is with us in our suffering, a constant presence, as close as our breath, His heart breaking for us, until one day when we see Him face-to-face.

About the Author

Benjamin Rattray is a newborn critical care physician in North Carolina where he serves as Associate Medical Director of Neonatal Intensive Care at the Cone Health Women's and Children's Center. He completed a pediatric residency and a neonatal-perinatal medicine fellowship at Duke University Medical Center, holds an MBA from LSU Shreveport, and is a Certified Physician Executive. He lives with his wife, three children, and a Golden Retriever in Greensboro, North Carolina.

Made in United States
North Haven, CT
08 December 2021

12184838R00096